Stretching
for Beginners

Published by Callisto Publishing LLC C/O Sourcebooks LLC
P.O. Box 4410, Naperville, Illinois 60567-4410
(630) 961-3900
callistopublishing.com

Printed and bound in China
WKT 2

Stretching
for Beginners

Improve Flexibility and Relieve Aches and Pains

with 75 Exercises and 24 Simple Routines

Natasha Diamond-Walker and Philip Striano, DC

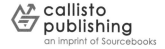
callisto
publishing
an imprint of Sourcebooks

I dedicate this book to my elegant mentor, Don Martin who has always encouraged me to stretch better and more.

Natasha Diamond-Walker

To Audra Avizienis, my gracious and tenacious editor who made this book possible.

Philip Striano, DC

CONTENTS

INTRODUCTION

"Movement is life." I first heard these words spoken by an old-school chiropractic professor during my first semester in graduate school. Over the years, these words have taken greater meaning for me—as a doctor practicing physical medicine and as an amateur athlete. Treating patients who suffer from aches and pains on a daily basis has reinforced the importance of movement in my professional and personal life. What I have discovered through my 25 years of experience is that the means to living an active, pain-free, and productive life is through appropriate and focused stretching. By stretching regularly, you can achieve a happier, well-balanced life.

For some time now, I've listened to my patients describe their experiences with chronic pain, as they go about the regular activities of daily life—painfully getting out of bed in the morning, feeling discomfort as they get in and out of their cars, straining their shoulders and backs at their desks for extended periods of time, and dealing with stiff necks and hands from constant texting. Many of these chronic conditions result from the modern sedentary lifestyle. I have come to the realization that stretching is the safest, most convenient, and most economical form of exercise that everyone can perform to improve their overall physical health. Along with greater health and fitness comes emotional well-being as well.

Stretching for Beginners is a fantastic resource for people of all levels of fitness. The detailed descriptions and illustrations of each exercise show you how to stretch the specific targeted muscles safely and effectively. Whether you are learning to stretch for the first time, beginning a new fitness routine, or recovering from an injury or illness, this easy-to-use book will help you achieve your goals by increasing your flexibility and decreasing pain and soreness.

My goal with this book is to provide you with a platform to improve your quality of life and physical health through the use of effective stretching. In part 1, you'll learn about the benefits of stretching, the science behind it, and how to perform stretches safely. Discover proper breathing techniques and how to incorporate stretching into your daily routines. If you want to jump right in, turn to part 1, chapter 3 (on page 17).

With so many different types of stretching techniques saturating the media, I wanted to keep things simple in this book. So I have limited the scope of stretches to four basic types: Dynamic or static, meaning with or without movement, and either passive or active, meaning with or without external force. Static stretching is probably the most common type and what most people think of when referring to stretching, such as touching your toes and holding the position.

In part 2 of this book, you'll find 70 essential stretches that are organized by different anatomical regions, denoting the focused muscles for each stretch. Each chapter focuses on a specific region of your body: From your neck to your core down to your feet. A brief synopsis explains the benefits of each exercise, including the types of activities or ailments that the stretch benefits the most. Each stretch also includes step-by-step instructions, accompanied by a clear illustration to help you perform the stretches properly. Once you're familiar with the stretches, you can try out the routines in part 3. You'll find routines for everyday stretching, for targeted ailments, and for specific sports.

Be smart before you start: As with any new exercise regimen, check with your physician before you begin, and perform a self-assessment. Be honest with yourself and realistic about your goals. If you progress gradually at a reasonable pace, you will see results. As a general rule of thumb: Stretch long, stretch slow, and stretch steady. Now get ready to begin the journey to a healthier new you.

—Philip Striano, DC

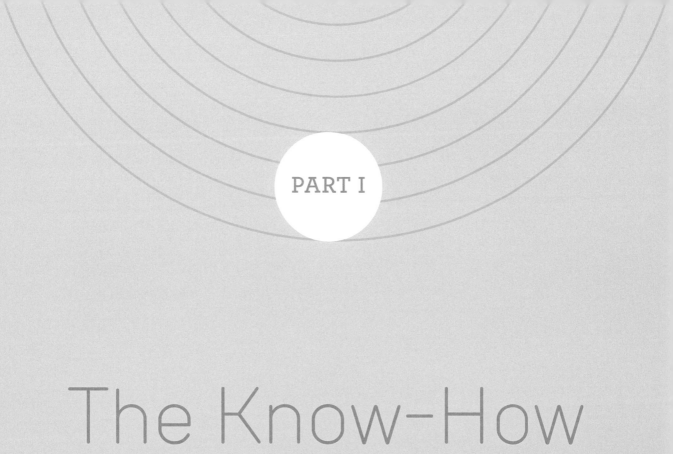

PART I

The Know-How

CHAPTER 1

WHY STRETCH?

Get up and stretch! The wonderful thing about stretching is that you really can perform it almost anytime and anywhere. Sitting at your desk too long? Get up and stretch. Feeling sluggish and stiff? Get up and stretch.

Stretching is one of the simplest and most rewarding exercises you can perform. A regular stretching routine can enhance your flexibility, muscle function, and circulation—all while calming your mind and improving your overall quality of life. Whether you're a couch potato, a fitness fanatic, or somewhere in between, you'll find that as you begin stretching regularly, you will move more fluidly and effortlessly.

For all of you beginners who envision having a more limber body, *Stretching for Beginners* can help you achieve your goal. One step at time, one stretch at time, you can turn your life around: Say good-bye to stiff muscles and creaking joints and say hello to a flexible body and a well-balanced life.

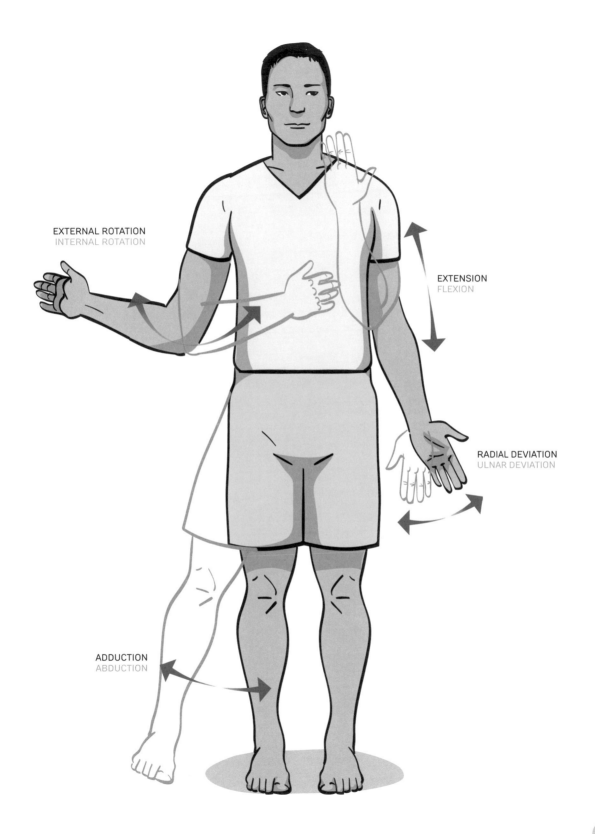

EXTERNAL ROTATION
INTERNAL ROTATION

EXTENSION
FLEXION

RADIAL DEVIATION
ULNAR DEVIATION

ADDUCTION
ABDUCTION

THE MUSCLES

The human body consists of three different types of muscles: cardiac, smooth, and skeletal. Cardiac muscle is unique to the heart, and smooth muscle surrounds the other internal organs; both of these muscle types are controlled involuntarily and are beyond the scope of this book. Skeletal muscles, on the other hand, are controlled voluntarily and are the most abundant muscles in the body. They're called *skeletal* muscles because they help secure the bones of your skeleton together. When you stretch for exercise, you're engaging your skeletal muscles.

What exactly happens to your muscles when you stretch them? Imagine a muscle as a telescoping pole or a collapsible umbrella: To lengthen the pole, you extend several interlocking segments; to shorten the pole, you collapse the segments into themselves. Muscles elongate and contract in a similar fashion. An individual muscle consists of bundles of muscle fibers, or large cells. These fibers are made up of cylindrical bundles of protein filaments called myosin and actin, which are arranged in stacked units of sarcomeres. Muscle contraction occurs as calcium ions trigger myosin and actin filaments to slide past each other, shortening the length of the sarcomeres much like a telescoping pole. As a muscle relaxes and elongates, the actin and myosin filaments slide apart, lengthening the sarcomere units.

It's important to remember that muscles don't move in isolation. Rather, when you move a muscle, you also move a bone and the respective joint. Generally speaking, muscles attach to tendons, which are the tough connective tissue between muscle and bone. Ligaments wrap around the joint and connect bone to bone, forming a capsule around the connection. Within a joint capsule is a viscous fluid that lubricates the bones. When you stretch a muscle, that muscle pulls on a bone and moves the respective joint. By stretching the appropriate muscles, therefore, you improve the range of motion in your joints. You also increase the blood flow to joint capsules, bringing more oxygen and nutrients to the area and keeping the muscles and joint healthier.

Muscle movements occur relative to their location on your body. A muscle attaches to a bone at an origin and an insertion point. The muscle origin serves as an anchor at a fixed attachment site, and the insertion is the movable part during a muscle contraction. A muscle pulls from the insertion site toward the origin of the muscle. In general, the origin of a muscle is the location closer to the body, relative to the insertion.

The direction of muscle movements is often described in oppositional pairs. The most basic of these are flexion and extension. Flexion is the movement at a joint that decreases the angle between the bones, whereas extension increases the angle between the bones. For example, as you bend your elbow to perform a bicep curl, you're flexing your muscles. As you straighten your elbow and lower your forearm, you are extending the joint.

Another directional pair consists of abduction and adduction. During abduction, a limb is moved away from the vertical centerline of the body, as when raising your leg out to the side. Adduction is the movement of a body part toward the vertical centerline. Rotation occurs either internally or externally along the long axis of a bone. If the rotation occurs toward the vertical midline of the body, the movement is internal. Conversely, if the movement occurs away from the vertical midline of the body, it is an external rotation. Finally, the oppositional pairs of pronation and supination describe turning a body part out or in, respectively, as when moving your foot.

Stretching for Beginners offers stretching exercises that target all the major muscle groups of the neck, shoulders, core, arms, and legs and incorporate all the basic muscle movements.

THE STUDIES

Your body was designed to move. Physiotherapists who study the effects of movement such as stretching invariably draw the same conclusion: Regular stretching of your muscles can vastly improve the quality of your life by increasing flexibility, boosting cardiovascular performance, and speeding up recovery from injuries. Here are just a few examples of some of the latest scientific research on stretching.

Greater Hamstring Flexibility

A 2016 study in the *Journal of Physical Therapy Science* reported that subjects who performed 15 minutes of self-myofascial release stretching for seven consecutive days increased their hamstring flexibility and hip proprioception.[1]

Stronger Heart Health

A 2019 study in the *Journal of Strength and Conditioning Research* indicates that stretching is an effective therapy for improving heart rate and cardiovascular health. Early research suggests that stretching enhances relaxation, baroreflex sensitivity, and nitric oxide bioavailability that may contribute to heart health.[2]

Better Balance in the Geriatric Population

A 10-week study published in the *International Journal of Health Sciences* in 2016 suggests that a lower-limb stretching protocol is effective in improving balance in the geriatric population, resulting in fewer falls and injuries. Sixty subjects participated in a regimen that included static stretching of the hip flexors, hamstrings, and gastrocnemius muscles for bouts of 30 seconds.[3]

Boosts Muscle Performance

A 2016 study in *MOJ Yoga and Physical Therapy* showed that young-adult athletes who performed dynamic stretching exercises such as butt kicks and straight leg kicks before more rigorous exercise increased muscle performance and power of their hamstrings and quadriceps.[4]

Enhanced Rehabilitation of Hamstring Injuries

Hamstring injuries are quite common in sports and other physical activities. In 2017, an eight-week study was conducted on dancers with hamstring injuries applying therapy based on static and active stretches, among other range-of-motion therapies. The results appeared in *The Journal of Sports Medicine and Physical Fitness* and indicate that stretching therapy helps reduce pain, increase flexibility, and improve muscle function.[5]

Improved Flexibility in Golf Players

A 2018 study in the *Journal of Exercise Physiology Online* examined the flexibility of 95 golfers during a season of golfing. The results indicate that stretch training improves the flexibility of golf players in their shoulders, lumbar spine, and ankles.[6]

THE BENEFITS

Regular stretching can enhance the quality of life for just about anyone—young or old, active or sedentary. Most people are aware that stretching improves flexibility and range of motion, but stretching has a lot more to offer. Stretching improves circulation, reduces muscle soreness and lower-back pain, prevents injuries, speeds up rehabilitation, decreases stress and aids sleep, improves posture and coordination, enhances athletic and sexual performance, and reduces age-related declines in physical fitness. Stretching has so many upsides and is a great complementary exercise to cardiovascular conditioning and strength training.

Increases Flexibility and Range of Motion

Stretching enhances flexibility so you can move through a full range of motion in your joints. Tight muscles and stiff joints can cause discomfort during everyday activities; for instance, shortened calf muscles or tight hip flexors can impinge on your ability to climb stairs. By elongating tight muscles and activating the associated joints, you can experience better overall mobility.

Reduces Pain and Injuries

Keeping your muscles and joints limber by stretching helps reduce your risk of injuries. If you don't keep your body supple, tiny microtears in your muscles can end up causing greater damage and lead to pain and injury. Muscles fibers can develop fibrotic adhesions, which prohibit the muscle from properly elongating (imagine a kink along the telescoping mechanism of muscle filaments). You're much less likely to pull a muscle during a sudden movement if you're flexible. This is especially true for athletes such as soccer or tennis players.

Speeds Recovery

After an injury or surgery, the affected area may be immobilized for a time. The lack of use and the build-up of collagen leads to a tightening of the muscles. Stretching helps soften the cross-fiber formation of scar tissue so the muscle tissue can be restored to normal function.

Boosts Circulation

When muscles contract and relax, they're working like a vascular pump. It's similar to squeezing a sponge: When you squeeze a wet sponge, it releases fluids; when the sponge is relaxed, fluid enters back into the sponge. Similarly, by stretching your muscles fully, you allow the blood to flow through the belly of the muscle and lubricate the entire joint. Blood flow nourishes the muscle tissue with oxygen and nutrients that are vital to the health and performance of the muscle. The fluid then carries away metabolic waste that was created by muscle use. A properly stretched muscle has an appropriate amount of blood flow going through it, which helps reduce stress on the related joint and may prevent undue wear and tear.

Remedies a Sedentary Lifestyle

The modern lifestyle often demands long hours either sitting at your desk or standing on your feet. The lack of normal movement is deleterious to proper functioning of muscles and joints. Various neck, shoulder, and back ailments can be traced to this way of life. Similarly, modern entertainment—for instance, watching TV or playing video games—also contributes to chronic fatigue. A targeted stretching routine could help counteract the effects of long periods of sitting or standing in one place.

Before or After a Workout?

The overall benefits of stretching are clear, but does it matter when you stretch? Much debate swirls around the benefits of stretching before or after vigorous exercise.

Before a strenuous workout, you should warm up your muscles with dynamic stretches that mimic the general movements of your workout. The idea is to get your blood flowing to your muscles to prime them for exertion. If you neglect to stretch, you risk exacerbating even the slightest muscle tear. Think of the blood in your body as the oil in your car's engine: You need to lubricate your muscles and joints before a workout just as an engine needs to warm up before it can function properly. Increased blood flow to your muscles allows for better, more efficient, and safer movements.

Performing static stretches after a rigorous workout, when the muscles are warm and flexible, improves their stretchability and, ultimately, their range of motion.

Improves Posture and Reduces Lower-Back Pain

From a biomechanical point of view, if muscles are too contracted at rest, they can affect postural alignment and cause pain along the spinal column. For instance, you could remedy slouched shoulders by elongating the pectoral muscles in the chest. Chronic back pain is often associated with limited flexibility in the hips and abnormally contracted hamstrings. Proper stretching of these areas could mitigate back pain.

Relaxes the Body and Improves Sleep

Stretching has a soothing effect on the body and the mind, and thereby helps to alleviate stress. The stimulation of stretch receptors in the muscles likely play a role in the relaxing effect of stretching exercises. When you're more relaxed, you're also more likely to sleep well.

CHAPTER
2

HOW TO STRETCH

Stretching is one of the easiest forms of exercise to learn. Just about anyone at any age and any level of fitness can reap the benefits from a new stretching routine. Follow these few simple guidelines on safety and proper technique, and you'll be ready to launch into your new fitness program.

WHAT MAKES A GOOD STRETCH?

Perform a Personal Assessment

When you venture into a new stretching program, you're likely doing it with a specific goal in mind. Whether you hope to improve your flexibility, your posture, or your overall health, the last thing you want to do is cause an injury that halts your efforts. The first step, therefore, before embarking on a stretching regimen is to assess your current physical condition. Be sure to have a physician's approval if you have any serious underlying conditions such heart disease or arthritis. Also be honest with yourself and perform a self-evaluation: Which are the most dysfunctional areas of your body in terms of patterns of motion? Where are your greatest weaknesses? First, address the major muscle groups that are affected, then target specific muscles within those larger groups.

Do a Reality Check

If you don't feel a little bit of discomfort, you're probably not stretching. Learn to listen to the signals that your body is giving you and understand your limits.

Set Realistic Goals

You are probably not a professional athlete, so be patient. Set modest goals for yourself over a period of time. For example, let's say you'd like to be able to touch your toes comfortably but you can only reach your knees right now. Aim for reaching the middle of shins in a few weeks, and acknowledge your small achievements. Think of this as a marathon, not a sprint. Go slow and steady.

Warm Up

Once you're ready to begin your first stretching exercise, you should make sure that your muscles are warm. For instance, don't stretch the minute you wake up when your muscles are still cold. If your muscles are not well lubricated yet, it's not a good time to stretch. Everybody gets microtears in their muscles from simple movements, and if you exercise when your muscles are cold, a small microtear could turn into more serious damage. If you'd like to stretch in the morning, take a hot shower to get your blood flowing before you start stretching.

Hold for the Correct Duration

For a stretch to be effective, you should hold the position for a minimum of 15 to 30 seconds. For the older population, some studies indicate a greater benefit when holding the stretch longer, for 30 to 60 seconds. As long as you don't feel light-headed, you can hold the stretch for up to a minute.

Breathe!

This may seem obvious, but if you're concentrating too hard on reaching a certain position, you make forget to take a breath. If you don't breathe while stretching, you will experience a decrease in oxygen to your brain, which could cause you to feel light-headed or pass out. Try to inhale and exhale slowly and deeply for the duration of the stretch; breathe continuously.

Find the Right Frequency

Begin stretching three to four times a week for several weeks. Gradually, increase the frequency as you progress and as your body adapts. Listen to your body: Your body will speak to you. If something hurts, stop. You should learn to recognize the difference between mild discomfort and frank pain.

Be Consistent

Find a time in your schedule every day or two to be able to give each stretch its appropriate effort and requirements. Keep in mind that it's better to do fewer stretches properly than to do too many in a rush.

Aim for Correct Form

Generally speaking, stretch with a long, slow, progressive focus on the muscles to produce a proper stretch. Any sudden jerky movements can result in injury or pain. A lot of novices tend to bounce through a stretch, which is counterproductive. If you bounce, you don't give your muscles a chance to work on a cellular, neurological, or chemical level. You need to allow enough time for a neurological response to relax the muscle.

TYPES OF STRETCHES

Starting a new stretching regimen can be daunting. The abundance of trendy exercise books and newfangled stretching methods can confuse people to the point of giving up before they've begun. *Stretching for Beginners* distills the vast options down to the bare essentials.

First of all, most basic stretches fall into just two categories: They are either dynamic or static, depending on whether or not you're moving during the stretch. Static exercises are further distinguished between passive or active, depending on whether an external force is applied to the targeted muscle. Other more sophisticated types of stretches—such as isometric and PNF—are essentially variations of these basic types of stretches and only a few are included in this book. Once you're more advanced, you can explore some of these more complex methods.

Two other types of stretching are worth mentioning here: myofascial release (MFR) and ballistic stretching. MFR essentially entails applying a stretch along the connective tissue, or fascia, between two areas of tension. It is often associated with the use of a foam roller to relax muscles and improve circulation, especially after a rigorous workout. This method is somewhat reminiscent of trigger-point massage therapy.

Ballistic stretching has largely fallen out of favor. Often confused with dynamic stretching, ballistic stretching involves bouncing through a movement beyond your maximum comfort zone. Imagine reaching down to touch your toes and bouncing down to get farther into the stretch. This approach is considered to be ineffective since your muscles don't have time to relax, and it's potentially harmful because pushing your muscles beyond their limit can easily lead to a tear. For these reasons, you would be wise to avoid ballistic stretching altogether.

Below you'll find the various types of stretches that are most relevant and productive for the beginner. Familiarize yourself with these methods so you have a better understanding of how to apply them to your new stretching routine.

Static and Dynamic

A static stretch involves holding a position for a specific duration, usually between 15 and 30 seconds. A dynamic stretch, on the other hand, requires continuous movement of your muscles. To illustrate the difference, let's consider a couple of wrist stretches. In the Wrist Flexor stretch (see figure, above right), when you flex your wrist and hold that position, you're performing a static stretch. Now make a fist and rotate your wrist in a continuous circular motion— that's the dynamic Fist Rotation stretch. Both static and dynamic stretches (see figure, below right) serve to improve your circulation, range of motion, and muscle flexibility.

WRIST FLEXION
PAGE 92

TYPE
STATIC, PASSIVE

You can perform dynamic stretches anytime. They get your blood flowing and are an invigorating way to start your day. Static stretches, however, are best performed when your muscles are sufficiently warmed up. So if you would like to do a series of static stretches first thing in the morning, for instance, consider warming up with some dynamic stretches or even taking a hot shower beforehand.

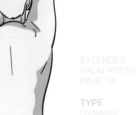

EXTENDED
PALM PRESS
PAGE 78

TYPE
DYNAMIC

Active and Passive

Static stretches are often grouped into two subcategories: active and passive. The most basic stretches are generally active stretches, meaning you are actively engaging the muscle without assistance from other sources. Passive stretches are those in which an external force is applied to a relaxed muscle. To illustrate the difference, let's go back to the examples of wrist stretches. The Wrist Flexor stretch is an active stretch because your wrist muscles are actively moving into the flexed position. Now if you were to relax your wrist and then use your other hand to bend your wrist and hold it in that position, that movement becomes a passive stretch. Both stretches are effective, but passive stretches allow for a more intense stretch.

Isometric and PNF

Isometric stretching is one of the quickest ways to improve your flexibility and strength. It involves contracting a stretched muscle as you resist against an outside force. The idea behind isometric stretching is that the external force equals the muscle resistance, so there's no movement—just steady pressure. (Isometric means "equal measure"). One way to achieve this type of stretch is by using the force of your own limbs. A perfect example of an isometric stretch is the yoga pose Prayer Hands (see page 98). By pressing your hands together at your chest, you're exerting equal pressure from both hands while your hands remain stationary. Because isometric stretches are a more advanced form of exercise, however, few appear in this book.

Proprioceptive neuromuscular facilitation (PNF) is another sophisticated method of stretching that is actually a combination of passive and isometric stretching. Originally developed as a rehabilitative exercise for stroke victims, PNF entails a cycle of first passively stretching a muscle by using an external force, then resisting against the force by contracting the muscle. When the pressure is released, the muscle relaxes and the range of motion increases. Performed correctly, the stretch becomes progressively more intense. This is the quickest way to increase flexibility, but it's also the most complex and is best performed with a knowledgeable partner.

Warm Up and Cool Down

If you're incorporating stretching into a more vigorous workout, dynamic stretches are preferred at the beginning of your routine, and static stretches are more appropriate for cooling down after a workout.

Dynamic stretches often mimic the movements of a workout, as in the High Knee Walking (see page 142), thereby targeting the appropriate muscle groups for that exercise. A runner, for instance, might warm up with High Knee Walking before heading out for a jog. After the run, the Hamstring Stretch would be a great way to loosen the leg muscles to maintain flexibility and reduce muscle soreness. If you would like to stretch a particularly tight muscle before a workout, you can perform a static stretch—just be sure to be sufficiently warmed up first.

PROPS

Props lend an extra dimension to stretching. You can better isolate a hard-to-reach muscle and intensify a stretch with the help of a prop. *Stretching for Beginners* introduces you to a few basic props—namely, resistance bands, small weighted balls, and large fitness balls. For the stretches that you perform on the floor, a yoga mat would provide a little traction and support, though it's not essential. In a pinch, you could also use household items in place of props. For instance, if you don't have a resistance band, you could try using a rolled-up towel instead. A folded blanket might come in handy if you need a little extra support under your hips. Once you get started on your stretching routine, you'll soon know what kind of props work best for you.

BREATHING AND COUNTING

One of the biggest mistakes that novices make when they first begin stretching is holding their breath: They focus so intently on getting the movement just right that they forget to breathe. Proper breathing, however, is an essential part of stretching. It improves circulation and keeps oxygen flowing through the body's cells, and it relaxes the muscles.

As you prepare for each exercise, inhale deeply into your abdomen rather than shallowly into the top of your lungs. Try to inhale through your nose in order to cleanse and warm the air for your lungs. As you begin to stretch, exhale in a slow, relaxed manner.

Remember to count too. At first, you may want to set a timer to get a sense of what 15 seconds feels like compared with 30 seconds. Some people like to count the seconds in their head; others prefer counting breaths. More advanced practitioners simply intuit the correct duration from past experience. With time, you'll find the counting method that best suits your style.

FAQ: Five Stretching Myths

1 If you're flexible, you don't need to stretch.

Someone who is naturally flexible may still have a few areas of tightness or some muscle imbalances. And flexibility isn't forever: As we age, we lose mobility. Starting healthy stretching routines early on will set you up for a higher quality of life in your later years.

2 You have to be flexible to stretch.

It doesn't matter if your range of motion is less than stellar—what matters is getting started. As long as you proceed slowly, you'll reap all the benefits and avoid getting injured.

3 No pain no gain?

Not true. Although a stretch should challenge your muscles, you should take care not to overstretch them. If your muscles are not properly warmed up before you stretch, you can cause tears that set you back days or even weeks while you heal.

4 You shouldn't stretch before a strenuous workout.

Your best bet is to perform dynamic stretches to boost your circulation and warm up your muscles before you exercise. Static stretches before a workout may actually impede performance by loosening your muscles too much. Save the static stretches for after your workout.

5 I'm too old for stretching.

On the contrary, stretching is essential for the more mature population. It improves the range of motion in your joints, especially your hips, and helps to prevent pain, stiffness, and injury. Stretching also enhances your sense of balance.

GETTING STARTED

You can do this! Start your new stretching routine today, even if you perform only one stretch. Whether you're young or old, with just a little bit of effort, you can quickly reap the many rewards of stretching—you will enjoy greater mobility, better posture, reduced stress, and an overall improvement in the quality of your life. With so much to gain, there really is no reason to delay any longer.

One of the great advantages of stretching over other forms of exercise is that you don't need expensive equipment or fancy workout clothes. All you need is a quiet, comfortable spot in your home or office where you set aside a few minutes every day to relax and decompress. Whether you prefer to stretch early in the morning, during your lunch break, or before going to bed—anytime that you can squeeze a few minutes out of your schedule will work just fine. No more excuses—get up and stretch!

HOW TO USE THIS BOOK

Stretching for Beginners is easy to use with clear illustrations and simple instructions on how to perform the exercises. Part 1 is essentially the brains behind the book. Here you'll learn about the basics of stretching. If you're curious about the dynamics of how muscles work—from the cellular level to joint structure—refer to page 4. If you still need a little convincing to begin your stretching routine, go to the Benefits section on page 7 to discover how regular stretching can improve your quality of life. There's also a section on the latest physiological studies that showcases the most current data on the many positive effects of stretching (see page 6 & 188).

Part 2 is the meat of the book, where you'll find 70 beginner stretches with detailed descriptions and illustrations of how to perform them. These six chapters walk you through the basic moves for every part of your body. Learn how to release tension in your neck (page 24), relieve stiffness in your back (page 42), alleviate tightness in your shoulders and chest (page 64), lengthen the muscles in your arms (page 88), improve mobility through your core and hips (page 108), and limber up your hardworking legs (page 132).

Once you've become comfortable with the basic exercises in part 2, you can move on to the routines in part 3. You'll find everyday routines like office stretches (page 166), routines that address specific aches and pains (page 170), and activity-related routines such as running and weight lifting (page 178). Everything you need to get you started is right here in this book.

LEVEL UP

For every beginner stretch in this book, you'll also find a description for an advanced variation. Take your time mastering the basic exercises before trying out these Level Up versions. Most importantly, listen to your body and remember that no two bodies are the same: A stretch that seems easy for one person may be too challenging for someone else. Similarly, if you're having difficulty with any of the basic stretches, you can simplify those as well. Modifications for certain stretches are offered in the Remember tips.

It will take time to master some of these Level Up stretches, so be patient and be kind to your body. A stretch shouldn't be painful. Yes, you do need to feel a bit of pressure while stretching to see results, but you should never push to the point of feeling pain. The benefits of stretching occur gradually over time.

Remember, your goal should not be about achieving perfect form on your first try; it's about doing the work and doing it regularly. Try to be consistent in your efforts and stretch at the same time every day so that you can build on your achievements and comfortably progress to a new level. When you commit to taking care of your body, that's when you begin to see some progress.

STRETCHING "ON THE FLY"

Stretching is probably the most versatile form of exercise you can practice. You can truly stretch just about anywhere. Exercises that are especially adaptable to a variety of venues have been labeled On the Fly throughout this book. In our modern sedentary lifestyle, we can really benefit from breaking up our daily routines and stretching our muscles to get the blood flowing and improve mobility.

At home, you would probably benefit from having a dedicated space where you perform your regular exercises. But even at home, when you're doing a chore such as preparing dinner, you can pause for a few moments and stretch your arms or wrists. If you work in an office at a desk all day, try to find time during your coffee break or lunch hour to ease any strain in your shoulders or back. And if you enjoy relaxing in front of the TV after a long day of work, instead of lying on the sofa, try sitting on the floor and stretching to counteract the stiffness in your joints and ease away any built-up tension.

For those of you who frequently travel for work, your entire body is probably begging for relief from the confined space of a car or an airplane. Try stretching out your neck or upper back while sitting on the plane, or if you're not shy, stand up in the aisle and do some simple arm and shoulder stretches. Who knows, maybe you'll start a trend. Wherever you are, you can work in a few moments of stretching. Your body will thank you.

PART II

The Stretches

QUICK OVERVIEW

These two illustrations show the areas of the body dealt with in this part of the book.

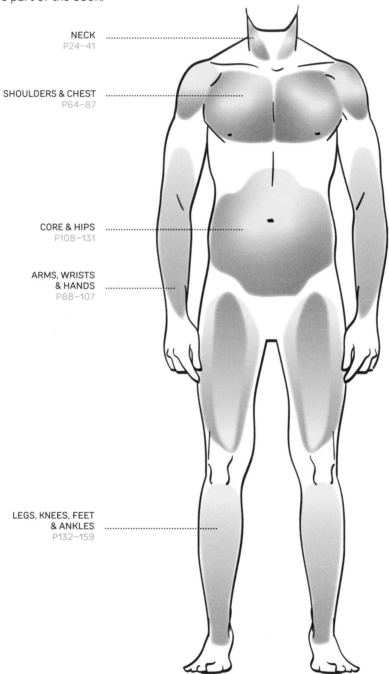

NECK
P24–41

SHOULDERS & CHEST
P64–87

CORE & HIPS
P108–131

ARMS, WRISTS
& HANDS
P88–107

LEGS, KNEES, FEET
& ANKLES
P132–159

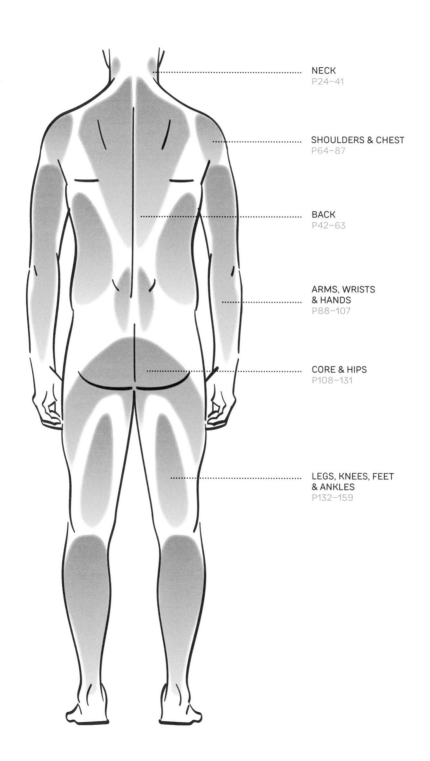

NECK
P24–41

SHOULDERS & CHEST
P64–87

BACK
P42–63

ARMS, WRISTS
& HANDS
P88–107

CORE & HIPS
P108–131

LEGS, KNEES, FEET
& ANKLES
P132–159

NECK

This chapter features nine neck stretches that improve the range of motion in your cervical spine, realign postural imbalances, and alleviate pain and stiffness. To regain the full range of motion in your neck, you need to target your muscles along all six planes of motion: forward flexion, backward extension, lateral flexion to the sides, and rotation to the sides. With greater mobility in your neck, you'll also enjoy deeper, more restful sleep as well as better overall function for longer periods of time.

NECK FLEXION

AFFECTED AREAS

Back of the neck: *levator scapula, splenius capitis*
Upper back: *upper trapezius*

GOOD FOR	LEVEL UP	ON THE FLY
This is a wonderful stress reducer that is effective in relaxing the neck muscles that are most often impacted by chronic tension.	When your neck is fully flexed, gently rotate your chin first to your left, then to your right to activate additional muscle fibers adjacent to the targeted muscles.	Take this stretch with you on the road. If you travel often for work and are prone to getting a stiff neck, try some neck flexion stretches to relieve the tension.

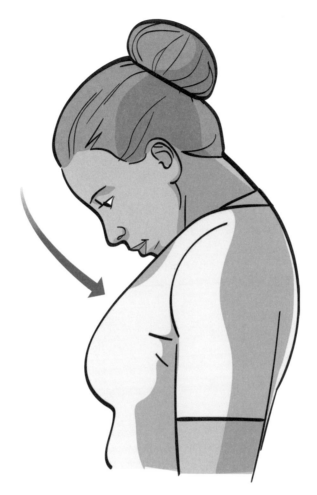

TYPE
STATIC, ACTIVE

INSTRUCTIONS

1   Stand in a neutral position with your feet shoulder-width apart or sit
    up straight in a chair with your hands loosely at your sides.

2   Inhale deeply to prepare, lengthen your spine, and loosen your
    shoulders.

3   As you slowly exhale, tilt your head downward, and try to touch your
    chin to your chest.

4   Hold for 15 seconds, continuing to breathe, and slowly return to the
    neutral position.

5   Perform three repetitions.

NECK FLEXION ASSISTED

AFFECTED AREAS

Back of the neck: *levator scapula, splenius capitis*
Upper back: *upper and middle trapezius*

GOOD FOR

This stress-prone area sometimes needs a little extra work to improve the range of motion in your neck and increase the blood flow—both arterial and venous. By applying gentle pressure with just your hands, you can greatly enhance the benefits of this stretch.

LEVEL UP

As you become more comfortable with this assisted stretch, add progressively more pressure to the top of your head and hold for up to 30 seconds.

REMEMBER

Continue to breathe throughout the stretch to ensure that oxygen is continuously flowing through your body. If you feel light-headed or dizzy during this stretch, take a break. Next time, reduce the amount of pressure you apply.

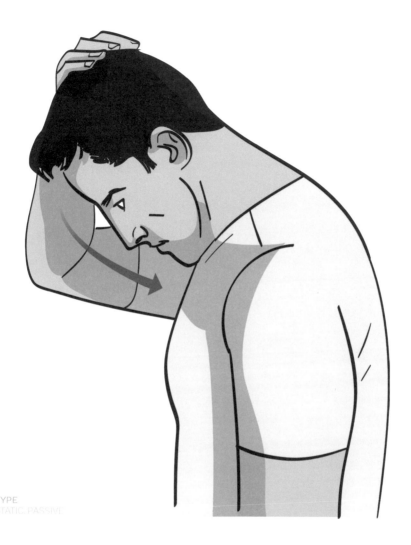

INSTRUCTIONS

1   Stand in a neutral position with your feet shoulder-width apart or sit up straight in a chair with your hands loosely at your sides.

2   Inhale deeply to prepare, and place a hand on the back of your head.

3   As you slowly exhale, gently press your head forward and downward just slightly beyond your unassisted range.

4   Hold for 15 seconds, and return to the neutral position.

5   Perform three repetitions.

NECK EXTENSION

AFFECTED AREAS
Front of neck: *platysma, sternocleidomastoid*

GOOD FOR
Modern-day devices such as cell phones, tablets, and laptop computers all require you to constantly look down, flexing your neck muscles. Prolonged habitual use of these devices can cause the cervical flexion muscles to become shorter, stronger, and tighter. This neck extension stretch offers the perfect movement to combat neck strain and rebalance the mobility in your neck.

LEVEL UP
Engage additional neck muscles by adding a twist. As you perform the exercise, slowly and gently rotate your chin to your right and hold for five seconds. Rotate to your left and hold for another five seconds.

REMEMBER
Be sure to keep your back straight and your shoulders down while performing this stretch so you don't cause undue strain in your neck. Never let the weight of your head fall back quickly.

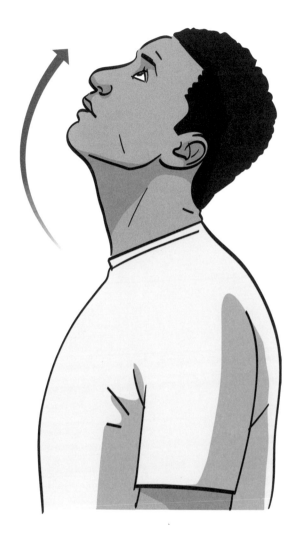

TYPE
STATIC ACTIVE

INSTRUCTIONS

1 Stand in a neutral position with your feet shoulder-width apart or sit up straight in a chair with your hands loosely at your sides.

2 Inhale deeply to prepare.

3 Slowly exhale as you lift your chin and extend your head backward.

4 Hold for 15 seconds, continuing to breathe, and slowly return to the neutral position.

5 Perform three repetitions.

NECK EXTENSION ASSISTED

AFFECTED AREAS

Front of neck: *platysma, sternocleidomastoid*

GOOD FOR

If you tend to sleep on your back with multiple pillows beneath your head, this stretch can help counteract some of the muscle imbalance you may have in your neck. This is an excellent stretch for anyone with a forward head posture.

LEVEL UP

To target more muscles fibers in the affected area, gently and smoothly rotate your chin to your right side and hold for five seconds. Then rotate your chin to the left and hold for another five seconds.

REMEMBER

Alternate the supporting hand with each repetition for a more balanced stretch through your neck. Go slow with this stretch so you don't strain your neck or shoulders.

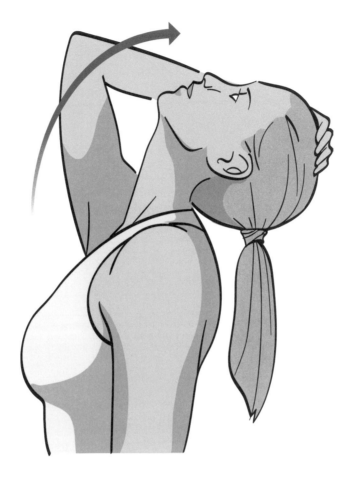

INSTRUCTIONS

1   Stand in a neutral position with your feet shoulder-width apart or sit up
straight in a chair with your hands loosely at your sides.

2   Inhale deeply to prepare, and place a hand on your forehead.

3   Slowly exhale as you lift your chin and gently push your head backward,
slightly beyond the point of your unassisted neck extension.

4   Hold for 15 to 20 seconds, continuing to breathe, and slowly return to
the neutral position.

5   Perform three repetitions.

NECK LATERAL FLEXION

AFFECTED AREAS

Sides of neck: *scalenes, levator scapula*

Upper back: *upper trapezius*

GOOD FOR

If you tend to sleep on your side, especially if you prop up your head with pillows, you may be putting unnecessary stress on your neck. This lateral stretch is highly beneficial for easing tension in the muscles along the sides of your cervical spine.

LEVEL UP

Ramp up the intensity of this stretch by stabilizing your torso while sitting in a sturdy chair. Hold onto the edge of the left side of the chair while bending your head to the right. Hold for up to 15 seconds and repeat on the opposite side.

REMEMBER

Concentrate on making sure the movement is emanating only from your neck. Don't lift your shoulders or bend at the middle of your spine.

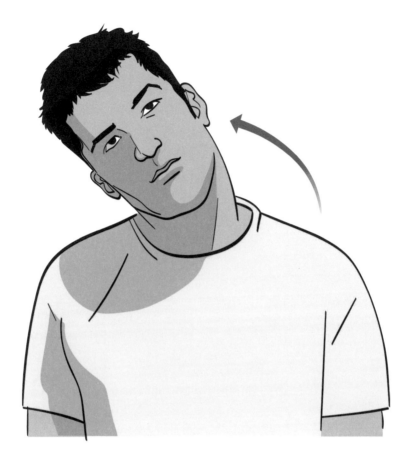

TYPE
STATIC, ACTIVE

INSTRUCTIONS

1   Stand in a neutral position with your feet shoulder-width apart or sit up straight in a chair with your hands loosely at your sides.

2   Inhale deeply to prepare.

3   Slowly exhale as you tilt your head to the right, as if to touch your ear to your shoulder.

4   Hold for 15 to 20 seconds, continuing to breathe, and return to the neutral position.

5   Repeat on the opposite side, and perform up to three times.

NECK LATERAL FLEXION ASSISTED

AFFECTED AREAS

Sides of neck: *scalenes evator scapula*
Upper back: *trapezius*

GOOD FOR

Chronic neck pain and stiffness can impair your daily function and impact your posture. Severe neck stiffness can also increase your risk of injury. By performing neck stretches regularly, you'll improve your range of motion and hold your head higher.

LEVEL UP

Activate some additional supporting muscles in your neck. As you perform the basic stretch, slowly lift your chin up and hold for five seconds. Next, tilt your chin down and hold there for another five seconds.

ON THE FLY

Unwind during your lunch break with this soothing stretch. It's a wonderful exercise to relieve neck and shoulder strain.

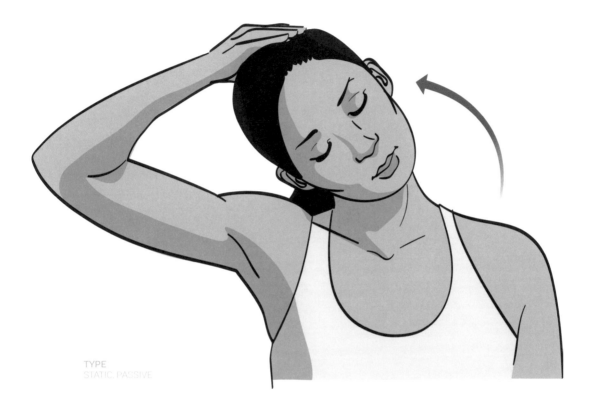

INSTRUCTIONS

1   Stand in a neutral position with your feet shoulder-width apart or sit up
    straight in a chair with your hands loosely at your sides.
2   Inhale deeply to prepare, and place your right hand on the left side of
    your head.
3   Slowly exhale as you tilt your head to the right, applying gentle force to
    the side of your head, pulling your ear toward your shoulder.
4   Hold for 15 to 20 seconds, continuing to breathe, and return to the
    neutral position.
5   Repeat on the opposite side, and perform up to three sets.

NECK ROTATION

AFFECTED AREAS

Neck: *sternocleidomastoid, levator scapula*
Upper back: *trapezius*

GOOD FOR

Make the roads safer by making your neck more mobile! If you have difficulty looking over your shoulder to make safe turns in your car, this is the stretch for you.

LEVEL UP

When your neck is fully rotated in the basic rotation, gently lift your chin and hold for five seconds, then lower your chin and hold for another five seconds.

REMEMBER

Find a rhythm to your breathing. Inhale while you're in the neutral starting position and exhale as you begin the stretch. Most importantly, keep breathing deeply throughout the exercise.

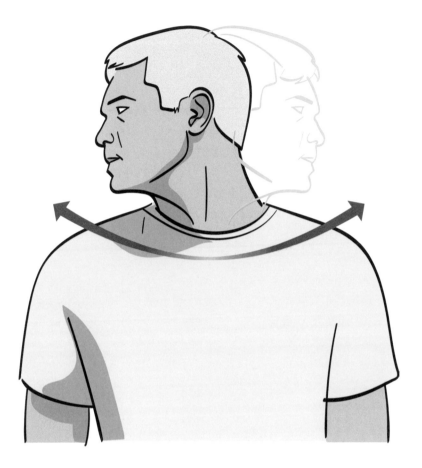

TYPE
STATIC, ACTIVE

INSTRUCTIONS

1   Stand in a neutral position with your feet shoulder-width apart or sit up straight in a chair with your hands loosely at your sides.

2   Inhale deeply to prepare as you lengthen your spine and drop your shoulders.

3   As you exhale, smoothly turn your head to the right and follow with your gaze over your shoulder.

4   Hold for 15 to 20 seconds, breathing deeply, and return to the neutral position.

5   Repeat on the opposite side, and perform three times.

NECK ROTATION ASSISTED

AFFECTED AREAS

Neck: *sternocleidomastoid, levator scapula, scalenes*
Upper back: *trapezius*

GOOD FOR

Sometimes if you can't perform a basic movement like turning your head, you might overcompensate with another part of your body such as your lower back. That can throw your alignment off-kilter and cause pain and stiffness. This exercise will help you regain some mobility in your neck and help prevent injury.

LEVEL UP

When you've advanced in this exercise, add a prop to assist with the movement and intensify the stretch. Wrap a resistance band around your head just above ear level and hold it with your right hand as you turn to your right. Hold for five seconds, and repeat on the opposite side.

REMEMBER

For a stretch to be effective, you should feel mild discomfort but never pain. When using props, be especially cautious so that you don't overstretch your muscles and cause an injury.

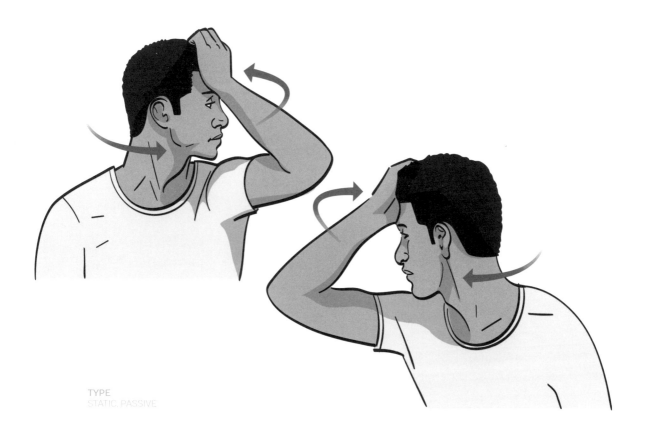

TYPE
STATIC, PASSIVE

INSTRUCTIONS

1   Stand in a neutral position with your feet shoulder-width apart or sit up straight in a chair with your hands loosely at your sides.

2   Inhale deeply to prepare as you lengthen your spine and drop your shoulders.

3   As you exhale, smoothly turn your head to the right and follow with your gaze over your shoulder.

4   When your neck is rotated as far as possible, place your right palm on your left temple and apply a smooth, gentle force slightly beyond your passive range of motion.

5   Hold for 15 to 20 seconds, breathing deeply, and return to the starting position.

6   Repeat on the opposite side, and perform three times.

CERVICAL STARS

AFFECTED AREAS
Entire neck: *sternocleidomastoid, scalenes, levator scapula, semispinalis*
Upper back: *trapezius*

GOOD FOR
Cervical Stars targets six planes of neck motion: flexing forward, extending backward, rotating left and right, and diagonal tilting to either side. This is a great exercise to perform for athletes to maintain the range of motion in their upper spine. Tennis players, golfers, and basketball players can benefit from this thorough neck stretch.

LEVEL UP
Gradually, intensify the stretch by holding for several seconds in each direction and using your hand to gently assist with the pressure.

REMEMBER
Always warm up your muscles before stretching. A hot shower in the morning is enough to get your blood flowing and get you ready for some exercise. Try waking up with a few reps of Cervical Stars while the hot water soothes your neck.

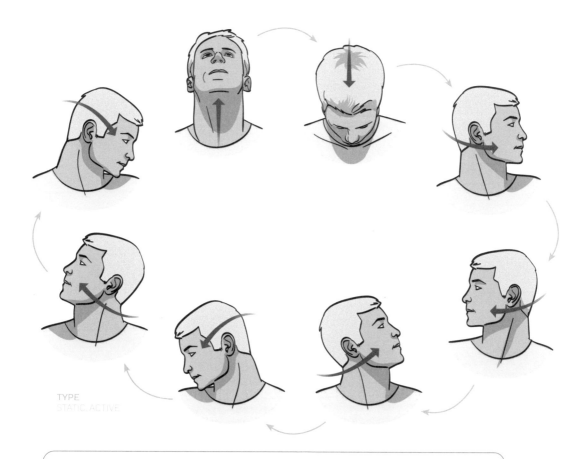

TYPE
STATIC, ACTIVE

INSTRUCTIONS

1 Stand in a neutral position with your feet shoulder-width apart or sit up straight in a chair with your hands loosely at your sides.

2 Imagine that there is a star shape in front of you with four intersecting lines: a vertical line, a horizontal line, and two diagonal lines.

3 Now imagine tracing those lines with the tip of your nose. Begin by slowly raising your chin up and lowering it toward your chest. Return to the neutral position.

4 Next gently turn your head to your left, then to your right. Return to neutral.

5 Raise your chin diagonally up and to your left, then down toward your right shoulder.

6 Finally raise your chin diagonally up and to your right, then down toward your left shoulder.

7 Return to the starting position, and repeat three times.

CHAPTER
5

BACK

Lower-back pain is one of the leading causes of work-related disabilities. Not only are the muscles of the back where we often carry stress, but they are also prone to injuries from lifting and twisting movements. Back stretches greatly improve the flexibility and resilience of your entire spine, from your neck to your tailbone.

CHILD'S POSE

AFFECTED AREAS

Lower back: *quadratus lumborum, erector spinae*
Middle back: *latissimus dorsi, lower trapezius, serratus anterior*

GOOD FOR

Child's Pose is an excellent stretch to loosen your entire spine, from your lower back all the way to your shoulders. Proper breathing during this stretch will also get your blood flowing.

LEVEL UP

Reach with your right arm under your chest so it's perpendicular to your left arm. Turn your torso slightly to your left to feel the deep stretch in your right shoulder. Hold for 30 seconds and repeat on the opposite side.

ON THE FLY

Deep inhalations and exhalations not only intensify this stretch but also increase your lung capacity and enhance oxygen circulation through your body.

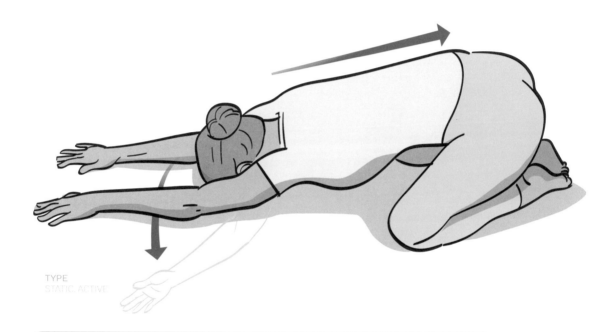

INSTRUCTIONS

1 Begin by kneeling on all four with your hands in line below your shoulders and your hips in line with your knees.

2 Inhale deeply to prepare, and slowly exhale while lowering your hips down to your heels.

3 Extend your arms straight ahead of you, sliding your hands forward.

4 Rest your forehead on the floor, and breathe deeply for 30 seconds.

5 Slowly rise up to the neutral position, and perform three repetitions.

CAT COW STRETCH

AFFECTED AREAS

Lower back: *quadratus lumborum, erector spinae*
Middle back: *latissimus dorsi, lower trapezius, serratus anterior*
Abdomen: *transverse abdominus*

GOOD FOR

A safe and simple beginner stretch, the Cat Cow is a full-body warm-up exercise. If you're looking for a great stretch to start off your morning, this yoga stretch is the one for you. It's also a wonderful way to release tension in your shoulders and find relief for lower-back pain.

LEVEL UP

Work on your balancing skills with this yoga variation called Tiger Pose. From the kneeling position on all fours, extend your right leg behind as you lift your head and chest upward. Next, curl your back as you bend your knee and bring your head downward. Gently touch your knee to your forehead. Repeat ten times per side.

REMEMBER

Move slowly through this stretch. As you curl your back, think of progressing one vertebra at a time, keeping your shoulders back and away from your ears.

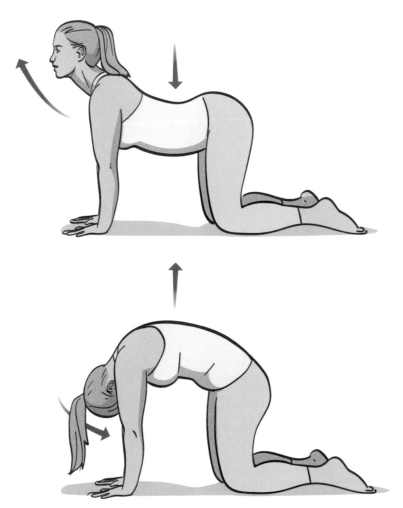

TYPE
DYNAMIC

INSTRUCTIONS

1 Begin by kneeling on all four with your hands in line below your shoulders and your hips in line with your knees. Lengthen your neck and roll your shoulders back.

2 Inhale and scoop your abdomen toward the floor, arching your back, and gaze forward.

3 As you exhale, tuck in your abdomen and slowly curl your back toward the ceiling while tucking in your chin toward your chest. Think of forming an upside-down U with your body.

4 Hold for a moment and inhale as you return to the neutral position.

5 Repeat 10 to 15 times.

DOOR-ASSISTED SIDE BEND

AFFECTED AREAS

Back: *latissimus dorsi, teres major, teres minor, erector spinae*
Abdomen: *abdominal obliques*

GOOD FOR

Many of us favor one side of our body and build tightness around overused muscles. This deep side bend lengthens the muscles in the middle of your back, one side at a time, so you can target the areas that need more flexibility.

LEVEL UP

Intensify the stretch by placing your hands higher on the doorframe. You'll engage more muscles all through the side of your body and along your spine.

ON THE FLY

This side bend is a very effective, deep stretch that you can perform anywhere you find a door.

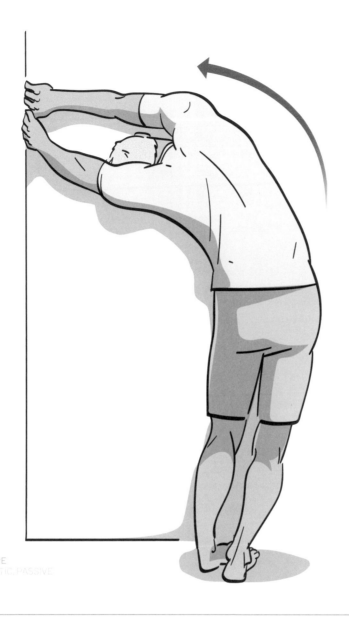

TYPE
STATIC, PASSIVE

INSTRUCTIONS

1. Stand straight with your feet together and about an arm's distance to the left of a doorframe.

2. Keeping your body facing forward, grab the edge of the doorframe with both hands, left over right, at about shoulder height.

3. Lean away from the doorframe, shifting your hips toward your left.

4. Hold for 30 to seconds and repeat three times per side.

WALL-ASSISTED UPPER-BACK STRETCH

AFFECTED AREAS

Upper back: *latissimus dorsi, trapezius*
Neck: *levator scapula, spelenius capitus*

GOOD FOR

Poor posture and slouching can often lead to upper-back pain, as can prolonged hours sitting at a desk or driving a car. This simple stretch targets the muscles in your upper and middle back, lengthening the muscles along your spine and releasing pressure between your shoulder blades.

LEVEL UP

Engage additional muscles along the sides of your neck by turning your head slowly to your right and holding for five seconds. Repeat to the opposite side.

REMEMBER

Imagine someone is trying to pull you away from the wall. Keep your back straight and try to lengthen through your arms and your spine as you lower your head and shoulders.

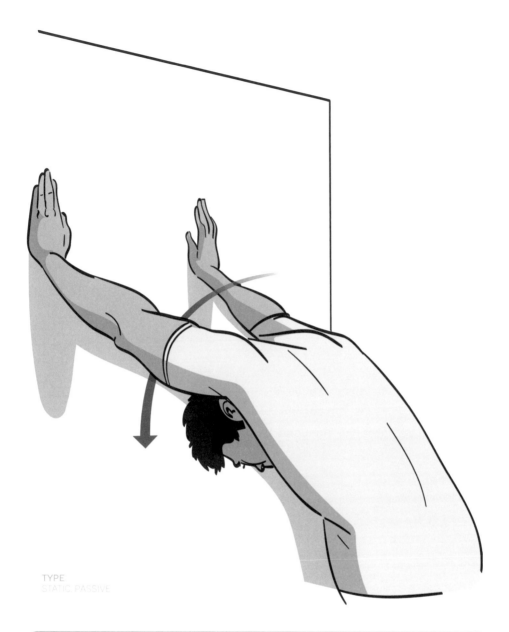

TYPE
STATIC PASSIVE

INSTRUCTIONS

1   Stand facing a wall with your feet hip-width apart.

2   Press your palms into the wall at shoulder height.

3   Step about two feet away from the wall.

4   Turn your gaze down at your feet and pull your shoulders away from the wall while pressing your hands firmly into the wall.

5   Hold for 30 seconds and repeat three to four times.

HEAD-TILTED FORWARD BEND

AFFECTED AREAS

Upper back: *trapezius*

Neck: *levator scapula, semispinalis, spelenius capitus*

GOOD FOR

Although it's not quite an inversion, by bowing your head in this stretch, you can feel that it really gets your blood flowing. This gentle stretch also soothes tightness in your upper back and is a good exercise for relieving daily stress.

LEVEL UP

Clasp your hands behind your back, rounding your shoulders, and perform the exercise as above. You'll feel a slightly deeper stretch in your upper back.

REMEMBER

During dynamic exercises such as this one, find a rhythm to your breathing. Move smoothly with each breath, lowering your head on exhale and raising your head on inhale.

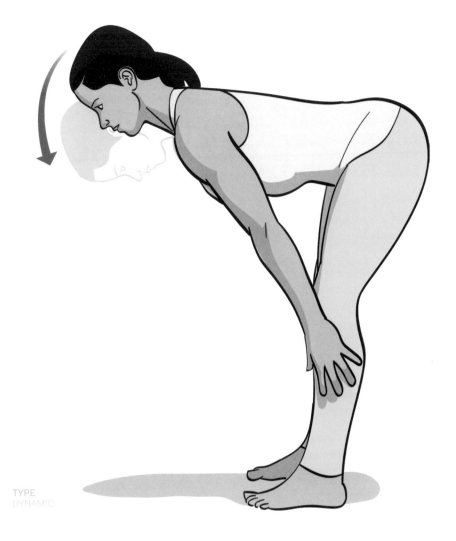

TYPE
DYNAMIC

INSTRUCTIONS

1   Stand straight with your feet hip-width apart.

2   Slowly bend forward from your hips and let your hands rest on your
    thighs just above your knees.

3   Inhale to prepare. Keeping your back straight, pull your shoulders down
    and back.

4   As you exhale, tilt your head downward, turning your gaze toward
    your knees.

5   Hold for a slow exhale, and slowly repeat the movement 10 to 20 times.

BEAR HUG

AFFECTED AREAS

Upper back: *rhomboids, trapezius*
Shoulders: *posterior deltoid*

GOOD FOR

Nothing like a bear hug to release tension and tight knots between your shoulder blades. This stretch may also alleviate the stiffness associated with bursitis and frozen shoulder.

LEVEL UP

Perform the Bear Hug as above, except tilt your chin into your chest and hold for 20 seconds. This extra movement will further lengthen the muscles running along your upper back.

ON THE FLY

When you're stuck on an airplane or a train and you feel tension building in your upper back, try this relaxing stretch to loosen up that space between your shoulder blades.

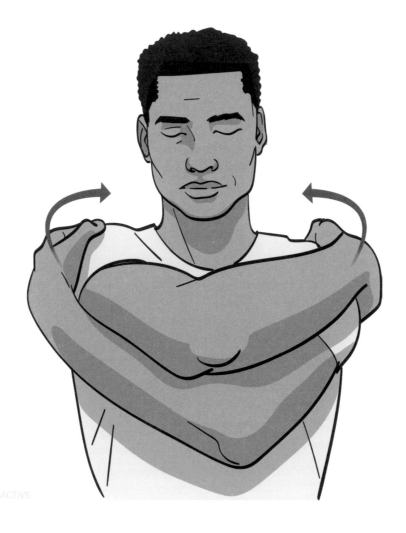

TYPE
STATIC, ACTIVE

INSTRUCTIONS

1 Stand straight in a comfortable stance.

2 Cross your arms in front of your chest, reaching your hands around your back and placing them on the opposite shoulder blade.

3 Press your hands into your shoulder blades and lift your elbows to shoulder height.

4 Pull your shoulders away from your body and hold for 20 to 30 seconds.

5 Release and cross your arms with the opposite arm on top and repeat twice per side.

QUADRUPED ROTATIONS

AFFECTED AREAS

Upper and middle back: *trapezius, latissimus dorsi*
Abdomen: *abdominal obliques*

GOOD FOR

Whenever you make a twisting movement in your torso, you're relying on the mobility of your thoracic spine in your upper and middle back. By targeting your T spine, this stretch helps to increase your range of motion in your daily activities—whether you're just reaching across a table, throwing a ball, or dancing the samba.

LEVEL UP

Perform the exercise as above, except as you raise your arm, sit back on your heels. This extra movement lengthens your spine as you rotate.

REMEMBER

Think of rotating your torso through your middle spine rather than twisting your joints. Don't use your elbow to swing through this stretch. Use a controlled motion and keep your hips stable.

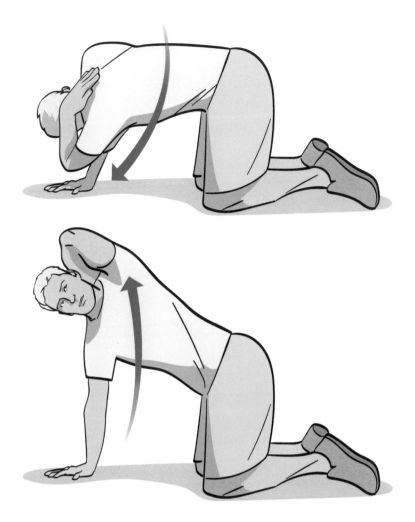

TYPE
DYNAMIC

INSTRUCTIONS

1 Begin kneeling on all fours with your hands in line with your shoulders and your knees in line with your hips.

2 Place your left hand behind your head and lift your elbow out to your side.

3 Inhale as you rotate through your thoracic spine and reach your left elbow down toward the floor, keeping your neck aligned with your spine and your hips stable.

4 As you exhale, slowly twist your torso up, readying your elbow toward the ceiling.

5 Perform this movement 10 times, and repeat three times on each side.

SINGLE KNEE TO CHEST

AFFECTED AREAS

Lower back: *quadratus lumborum, erector spinae*
Buttocks: *gluteus maximus*

GOOD FOR

This easy, soothing stretch releases tension and stiffness in your lower back. If you've been on your feet all day, you'll appreciate the relaxing position as you stretch open the spaces between your lower vertebrae and improve the circulation in your lower back.

LEVEL UP

Tuck a folded blanket or towel under your hips to increase the stretch through your lower spine. Flex your extended leg to engage your hamstrings.

REMEMBER

Keep your lower back pressed into the floor. If you feel pain in your back during this stretch, try keeping your knees bent throughout the exercise rather than extending one leg.

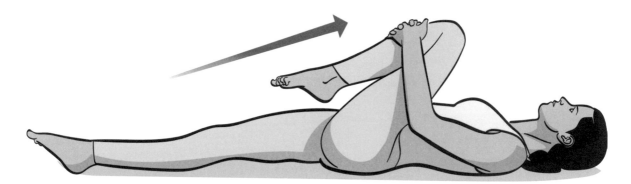

TYPE
STATIC-PASSIVE

INSTRUCTIONS

1 Lie on the floor with your knees bent.

2 Bring your left knee toward your chest and wrap your hands around
   your left shin just below your knee. Gently pull your knee closer
   into your chest.

3 Extend your right leg flat on the floor.

4 Hold for 15 to 20 seconds and return to the neutral position.

5 Repeat three times on each leg.

DOUBLE KNEE TO CHEST

AFFECTED AREAS

Lower back: *quadratus lumborum, erector spinae*
Buttocks: *gluteus maximus*

GOOD FOR

The Double Knee to Chest stretch is one of the gentlest yet most effective spinal decompression exercises you can do. As you curl your legs into your chest and roll your back down, you'll feel a soothing massage along your spinal column. This stretch works wonders for lower-back pain.

LEVEL UP

Try this rolling motion for a gentle spinal massage. Clasp your hands together behind your knees and slowly roll forward lifting one vertebra at a time off the floor. Gently roll back down.

REMEMBER

This stretch should be relaxing, not painful. If you have chronic lower-back pain, move slowly through this exercise so as not to aggravate your condition.

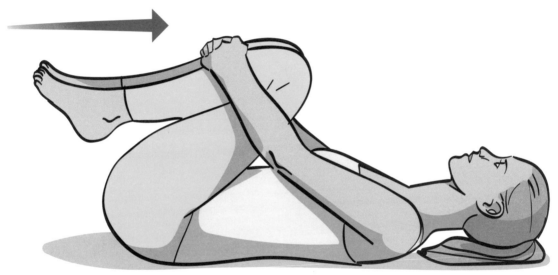

TYPE
STATIC, PASSIVE

INSTRUCTIONS

1   Lie on the floor with your knees bent.

2   Bring one leg at a time into your chest and wrap your hands around
    your shins just below your knees.

3   Gently pull your knees closer into your chest, and hold for 15 to
    20 seconds.

4   Return to the neutral position and repeat three times.

LOWER-BACK ROTATION

AFFECTED AREAS

Lower back: *quadratus lumborum, erector spinae*
Abdomen: *transverse abdominus, abdominal obliques*

GOOD FOR

Chronic lower-back pain is a major health issue in sedentary societies such as ours. Developing flexibility in your lower back, along your lumbar spine, can minimize pain and improve functional movement. A limber lower back also helps realign your posture and prevent injury.

LEVEL UP

Intensify the stretch by crossing your legs at your thighs and then dropping your knees to the side. You'll feel it in your lower back as well as your glutes.

ON THE FLY

Keep your knees pressed together to gain the most benefit from this stretch. If your knees keep separating, place a small rolled-up towel between your knees and squeeze them together.

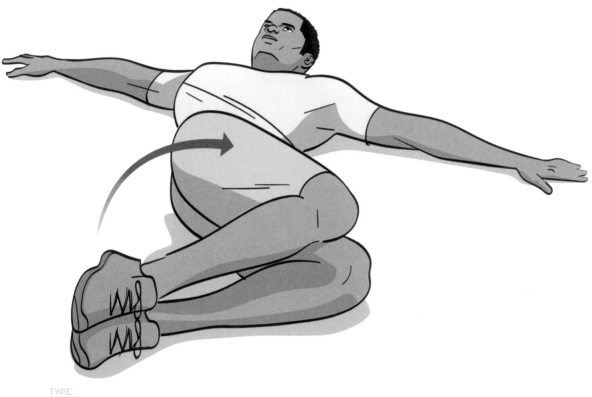

TYPE
DYNAMIC

INSTRUCTIONS

1   Lie on your back with your knees bent and your arms extended out to your sides with palms facing up.

2   Press your knees and feet together, and lower your knees to your left side as far as you can go without straining.

3   Keep your shoulders and arms pressed into the floor.

4   Hold for 20 to 30 seconds, return to neutral, and repeat on the opposite side.

OPEN BOOK STRETCH

AFFECTED AREAS

Middle back: *quadratus lumborum, erector spinae*
Buttocks: *gluteus medius*
Abdomen: *external obliques*

GOOD FOR

This chest opener helps you regain mobility in your middle back along your thoracic spine. If you tend to slouch and roll your shoulders forward, this stretch can help improve your postural alignment and loosen up tightness in your T spine.

LEVEL UP

Add a dynamic movement to this stretch. Lie on your side with knees bent, and press your left hand on your right thigh. Extend your right hand on the floor in line with your shoulders. Now open your right arm, lifting it straight overhead and over onto the floor on your right while extending your lower leg in line with your body. Hold for a few seconds, return to neutral, and repeat on the opposite side.

REMEMBER

As you twist your torso, try to touch both shoulders to the floor. Help your torso twist by pulling with the hand that's resting on your ribcage.

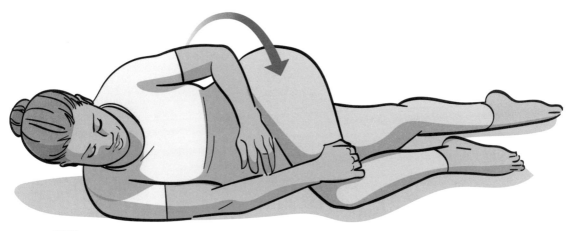

TYPE
STATIC, PASSIVE

INSTRUCTIONS

1 Lie on your right side with your knees bent and legs stacked on top of each other.

2 Press your right hand on your left thigh, and extend your lower leg in line with your body.

3 Place your left hand on your right ribcage and inhale to prepare.

4 Rotate your torso to your left as far as you can, and hold for 10 to 15 seconds.

5 Return to neutral and repeat three times on each side.

SHOULDERS & CHEST

Shoulders are often the repository of accumulated daily stress, tightening and rising up toward the ears. The chest, meanwhile, often becomes cramped and concave after spending hours working at a desk. The following stretches can help open both areas and restore proper posture.

POSTERIOR ARM CRADLE

AFFECTED AREAS
Front of shoulders: *anterior deltoids*
Chest: *pectorals*

GOOD FOR
This peaceful seated stretch eases strain in the front of your shoulders while opening your chest and lengthening your neck. If you're feeling stressed or simply longing to open the front of your body, this is the stretch for you.

LEVEL UP
For a deeper opening through your chest and lengthening along your spine, hold the stretch, and slowly tilt your head forward, bringing your chin into your chest. Slowly tilt your head backward, raising your forehead to the ceiling.

ON THE FLY
This stretch can be done at home, in the office, or while standing, which makes it a great on-the-move option.

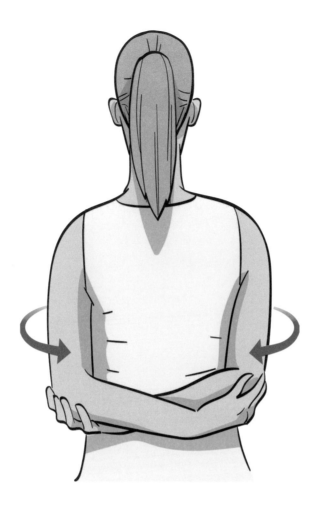

TYPE
STATIC-ACTIVE

INSTRUCTIONS

1   Find a comfortable place to sit, either on the floor or in a chair. Place your palms on your thighs and inhale.

2   Exhale as you push your shoulders down and roll them slightly back while lengthening your neck.

3   Gently bend your right arm behind your back and let it rest behind your hip. Bring your left hand behind your back to meet your right hand.

4   Slowly walk your hands in toward each other and up your forearms, settling at the opposite elbow.

5   Open your chest wide and breathe deeply and slowly for 30 to 45 seconds.

ARM STRETCH LYING DOWN

AFFECTED AREAS
Full body

GOOD FOR

Try this exercise if your core muscles are a bit lax or if you have habitual neck tension or less than perfect posture. Take a moment to get in touch with your body and feel the support of the hard surface beneath you.

LEVEL UP

Opt for a more expansive stretch through your body by opening your arms and legs wider. Knit your ribcage closed and press the middle of your back gently down into the floor beneath you. Breathe deeply here for 45 to 60 seconds.

REMEMBER

As much as you'd like to relax in this pose, keep your shoulders from creeping up toward your neck. Allow the top of your head to pull away from your chest to help create space along the back of your neck.

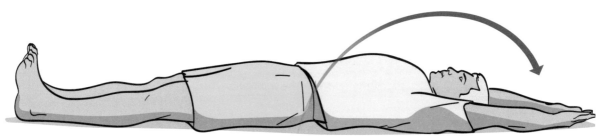

INSTRUCTIONS

1   Find an area, preferably a hard surface, where you can safely lie down with your arms and legs fully extended.

2   Lie down with your arms at your sides with your palms facing up. Keeping your arms on the floor, slowly extend your arms overhead and at a slight diagonal.

3   Slide your feet open to more than hip-width apart, forming an X with your body.

4   Create opposition in your stretch by imagining your arms and legs pulling away from your torso.

5   Hold for 30 to 60 seconds.

ARM CIRCLES

AFFECTED AREAS

Shoulders: *deltoids*

Upper back: *trapezius, rhomboids*

Rotator cuffs

GOOD FOR

Arm circles provide an opportunity to get your energy flowing while expanding a full range of movement that begins from inside the shoulder rotators. If you feel tight in your neck and shoulders, this dynamic stretch will help release pent-up tension in those areas.

LEVEL UP

For an added challenge and more expansion through your chest, sweep your arms around in larger circles. When you're more advanced, try holding light weights or use weighted wrist cuffs.

REMEMBER

Proper breathing during this exercise will give you greater results. Although this is a dynamic stretch, keep your torso steady and control the movement to prevent pulling a muscle.

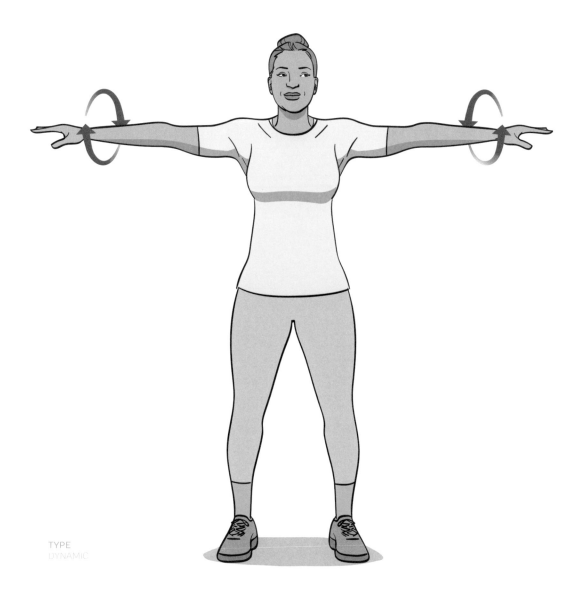

INSTRUCTIONS

1 Begin by standing with your feet hip-width apart and your arms hanging loosely at your sides.

2 In one graceful sweep, bring your arms up and out to your sides, keeping your elbows straight.

3 Slowly rotate your arms forward and circle them down and around, forming small circles.

4 Repeat a series of five circles, and repeat in the opposite direction.

WALL-ASSISTED CHEST OPENER

AFFECTED AREAS
Chest: *upper pectorals*
Front of shoulders: *anterior deltoids*

GOOD FOR
This wall-assisted stretch opens your chest and lengthens the muscles that wrap around your shoulders. Weightlifters who build up their pecs would benefit from this soothing stretch. It also helps improve postural imbalances such as rounded or hunched shoulders.

LEVEL UP
For a more intense chest opener, place your left forearm on the wall slightly to your left. You'll feel a deeper stretch as you turn your body away from the wall. Gaze over your right shoulder to extend the stretch through your neck.

REMEMBER
Engage your core muscles and root down through your legs as you stand at the wall, so that your weight is fully supported from your center.

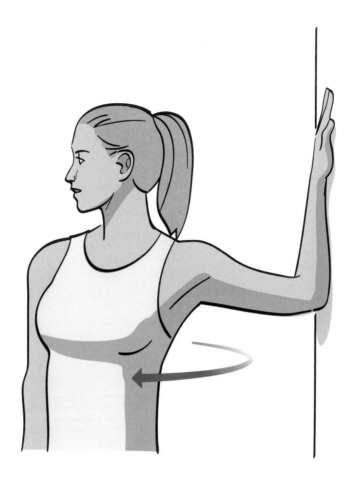

TYPE
STATIC, PASSIVE

INSTRUCTIONS

1   Stand facing a wall and about a foot away it with your feet hip-width apart.

2   Raise your left arm in front of you, bending your elbow to 90 degrees.

3   Rest your forearm and palm on the wall in front of you. Your elbow should be at the same height as your shoulder.

4   Shift your weight to your left foot as you step your right foot behind. Pivot your feet so that they are parallel to the wall and the left side of your body is facing the wall.

5   Press your left forearm into the wall as you turn your torso and head to your right.

6   Inhale and exhale deeply as you hold here for 15 to 30 seconds.

7   Switch sides and repeat three times.

BENT-ARM FLY

AFFECTED AREAS

Back of the shoulders: *posterior deltoids*

Chest: *pectorals*

Upper back: *trapezius*

Upper arms: *biceps*

GOOD FOR

The focus of this stretch is to align your hands, forearms, and biceps along the midline of your body. The opening and closing action of the movement shortens and expands your pectoral muscles while increasing mobility in your shoulders.

LEVEL UP

As your forearms touch, hold the position and slowly bow your head, tucking your chin into your chest between your arms. Inhale and exhale in this position for 15 to 30 seconds.

REMEMBER

Keep your elbows at shoulder height throughout the movement. If you are not able to touch your forearms together, simply bring your palms together at first, then gradually work toward pressing your forearms together.

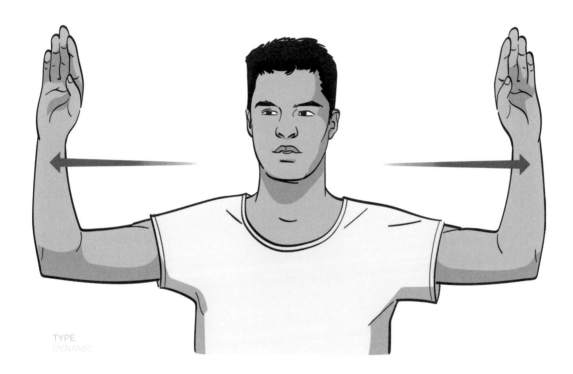

INSTRUCTIONS

1   Stand tall with your feet hip-width apart.

2   Open your arms straight out to your sides with your palms facing
    forward.

3   Bend your elbows, making a right angle with each arm so your fingers
    point toward the ceiling, and inhale.

4   Exhale as you bring your arms forward, and press your forearms
    together near your face.

5   Inhale with your arms together, and exhale as you open your arms.

6   Repeat 10 times.

ELBOW CIRCLES

AFFECTED AREAS

Shoulders: *deltoids*

Rotator cuffs

Chest: *pectorals*

Upper back: *trapezius*

GOOD FOR

This stretch targets all the muscles of your shoulders and is great for improving your range of motion. The circular movement of this exercise provides a nice warm-up for your upper body and also lengthens the sides of your torso.

LEVEL UP

Intensify the stretch by performing wider circles and by pressing your elbows together at the beginning of the stretch. Try to keep your elbows in contact as they pass in front of your chest in either direction.

REMEMBER

Pay close attention to the range of movement in each of your shoulders as you perform these circles. Very often one shoulder is tighter than the other. Strive for symmetrical movements on either side.

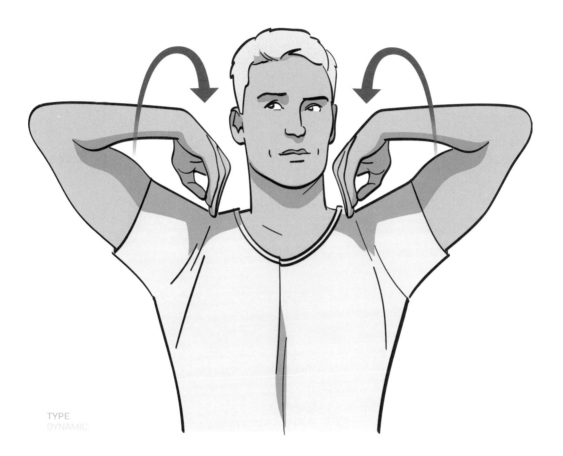

INSTRUCTIONS

1   Touch your fingertips to the tops of your shoulders, and wing open your elbows to your sides.

2   Move both arms in unison as you trace your elbows in small circles, first to the front, then up and back, then down and around to the front.

3   Perform 10 circles and repeat in the opposite direction.

HANDS CLASPED SHOULDER EXTENSION

AFFECTED AREAS

Front of shoulders: *anterior deltoids*

Chest: *pectorals*

GOOD FOR

Restore some shoulder flexibility and release tension in the front of your shoulders and chest. Stretching the anterior deltoids at the front of your shoulders is a great counterpoint to tight, slumped shoulders and helps improve your posture.

LEVEL UP

Deepen the stretch along the front of your neck and chest by pulling your clasped hands downward and away from your body as you tilt your chin up slightly. Hold for five seconds.

REMEMBER

The movement here is minimal—embrace the limit in this stretch and be gentle on yourself. Be careful not to strain your neck by tilting your head too far back.

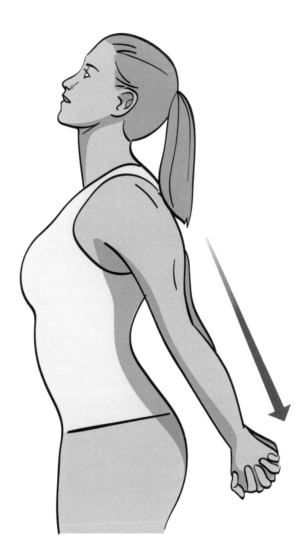

TYPE
STATIC, ACTIVE

INSTRUCTIONS

1   Stand tall with your feet about shoulder-width apart.
2   Elongate you neck, and pull your shoulders down and slightly back.
3   Reach behind you, and clasp your hands behind your back with your palms facing up.
4   Keeping your elbows straight, pull your hands away from your body to open your chest, and lengthen along the front of your shoulders.
5   Hold for 15 to 30 seconds, slowly release, and repeat three times.

EXTENDED PALM PRESS

AFFECTED AREAS

Upper back: *trapezius*

Shoulders: *deltoids*

Chest: *pectorals*

Wrists

GOOD FOR

Alleviate tension headaches, tight shoulders, and general stress that can affect your upper body. The Extended Palm Press helps ease tightness in your arms, neck, and shoulders as you move your hands along the vertical midline down the front of your body.

LEVEL UP

As your hands are interlaced at hip height, tilt your chin up slightly to feel more of a stretch along your chest. As you move your hands up above your head, allow your chin to fall into your chest to lengthen your upper-back muscles.

REMEMBER

If you are struggling with your balance during this stretch, have a seat and work through this stretch while sitting—it will be just as effective as if you were standing.

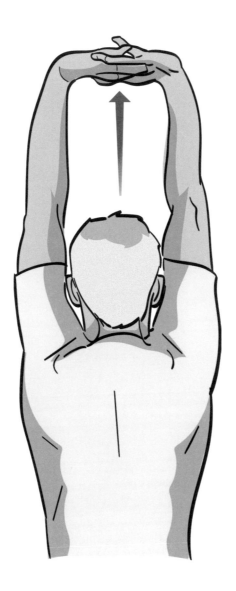

TYPE
DYNAMIC

INSTRUCTIONS

1   Stand in a neutral position with your feet shoulder-width apart or sit up straight in a chair with your hands loosely at your sides.

2   Inhale deeply to prepare.

3   Slowly exhale as you lift your chin and extend your head backward.

4   Hold for 15 seconds, continuing to breathe, and slowly return to the neutral position.

5   Perform three repetitions.

CRISSCROSS ARMS

AFFECTED AREAS
Chest: *pectorals*
Shoulders: *deltoids*
Upper back: *trapezius*

GOOD FOR

The swing in this stretch activates your pectorals in two ways: by extension when opening your arms, and by contraction when crossing. If you're looking for an energetic release for your upper body, this is the move for you.

LEVEL UP

For added mobility in your shoulder joints, pitch forward from the waist and look down. Shake your arms out in front of your legs, and perform the stretch while bent over. Allow gravity to lengthen your arms out and away from your shoulders.

REMEMBER

Take your time as you swing through the crisscross movement. You really need only a little force to get a good stretch; less is definitely more with this exercise.

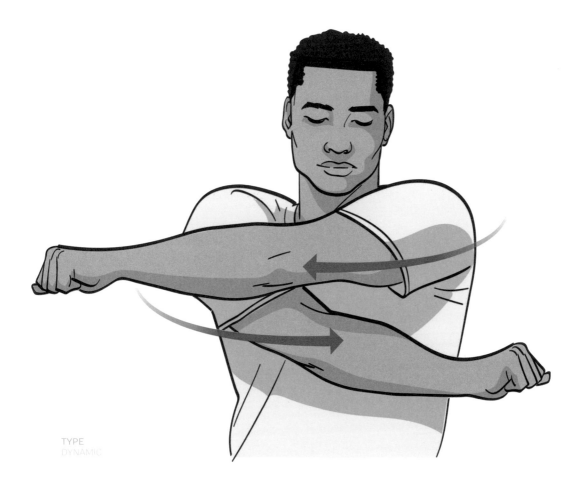

INSTRUCTIONS

1 Start by shaking your arms out loosely in front of you, then down at your sides.

2 Give yourself a big hug with your right arm above your left arm. Inhale and exhale.

3 With a smooth, controlled movement, swing your arms wide open to your sides, and swing them back in across your chest, left arm over right.

4 Continue alternating your arm position as you swing open and close.

5 Continue for 30 to 60 seconds.

SHOULDER HYPEREXTENSION

AFFECTED AREAS
Upper back: *trapezius*

Shoulders: *deltoids*

Forearms

Wrists

GOOD FOR
Performing repetitive tasks, whether at work or at home, often involves asymmetric movement patterns that can eventually cause parts of your body to hold tension and create discomfort. This elbow inversion relieves tightness around your shoulders and arms in a whole new way.

LEVEL UP
This move is already quite intense; however, if you'd like more of a challenge, make your hands into fists, and work toward bringing your fists to touch behind the middle of your back, then imagine bringing your elbows forward.

REMEMBER
As soon as you feel a stretch, at whatever point that is for you, stop there and breathe. Don't push too hard in this stretch.

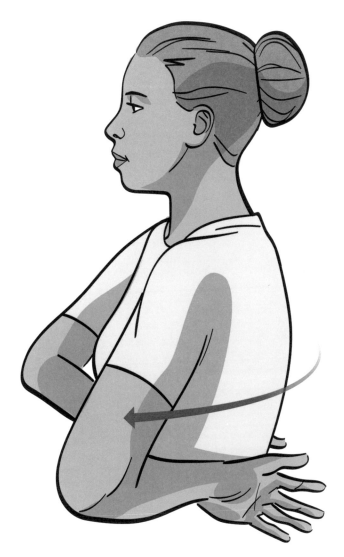

TYPE
STATIC, ACTIVE

INSTRUCTIONS

1 Find a comfortable position either standing or seated.

2 Lengthen your back, and place the tops of your hands high on
   your waist.

3 Slowly slide your fingers and wrists back behind your lower ribcage.

4 Gently rotate your shoulders and elbows forward. Elongate your neck,
   and keep your shoulders soft as your shoulders slide forward.

5 Hold for 30 to 60 seconds, and repeat three times.

SHOULDER CIRCLES

AFFECTED AREAS
Upper back: *trapezius*
Chest: *pectorals*
Shoulders: *deltoids*

GOOD FOR
Sometimes the smallest movements can have the greatest impact. When you have a moment of peace, close your eyes and allow this stretch to melt away pent-up tension in your upper body. Perform these shoulder circles as big or as small as you'd like.

LEVEL UP
Expand the stretch into the sides of your neck by isolating one shoulder at a time. Lean your right ear toward your right shoulder as you circle your left shoulder. Then lean your left ear toward your left shoulder as you circle your right shoulder.

ON THE FLY
This is a very effective stress-relieving stretch that can be done multiple times a day. And you can take it with you anywhere you go.

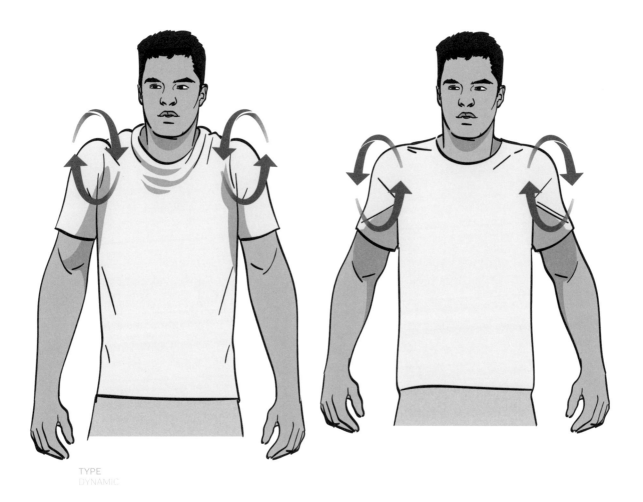

TYPE
DYNAMIC

INSTRUCTIONS

1   Stand straight with your feet about hip-width apart. Allow you arms to dangle loosely at your sides.

2   Breathe in, and focus your attention on your shoulders.

3   Shrug your shoulders up toward your ears, and circle them back and around to the front.

4   Repeat 10 times in each direction.

OPEN-DOOR PEC STRETCH

AFFECTED AREAS

Chest: *pectorals*

Shoulders: *deltoids*

Upper arms

GOOD FOR

This restorative chest opener helps counteract slumped shoulders and poor posture and is especially beneficial for the weight-lifting population. You'll feel your pectoral muscles lengthen and your shoulders relax as you gently push through this stretch.

LEVEL UP

Try one arm up at a time and add a twist. Place your left palm on the doorframe, and as you step your left foot forward, turn your head to the right. Hold for 30 seconds, and repeat on the opposite side.

ON THE FLY

This is an easy and convenient stretch to perform at the office on your lunch break or before a meeting.

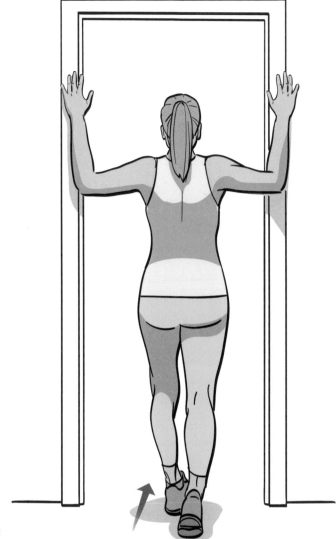

TYPE
STATIC, PASSIVE

INSTRUCTIONS

1. Stand in the middle of an open doorway with your feet hip-width apart.
2. Raise your arms, and rest your palms on either side of the doorframe. Your elbows should be in line with your shoulders.
3. Step forward slightly with one foot, and gently lean forward until you feel the stretch across your chest and shoulders.
4. Hold for 30 to 45 seconds, and repeat three times.

ARMS, WRISTS, & HANDS

The arms, along with the wrists and hands, are the versatile workhorses of the body—performing feats of physical strength and detailed maneuvers. Arm stretches also benefit the delicate mechanisms of the wrists and hands by strengthening them against injury and relieving stiffness and pain.

WALL-ASSISTED BICEP STRETCH

AFFECTED AREAS

Shoulders: *deltoids*

Chest: *upper pectorals*

Upper arms: *biceps*

Forearms: *brachialis*

GOOD FOR

This simple wall-assisted stretch lengthens the muscles along your chest, down your arms, and into your wrists. Find soothing relief from tight chest muscles and stiff shoulders and arms.

LEVEL UP

For a more intense opening along the back of your neck, slowly turn your head away from the wall to look toward the opposite shoulder.

REMEMBER

Root down through your legs and engage your core muscles so that your weight is fully supported from your center. Try not to tense up your shoulders.

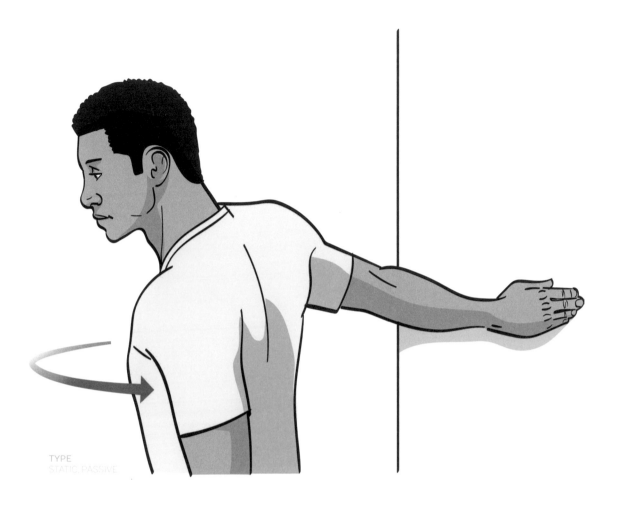

INSTRUCTIONS

1 Stand with your right side about a foot away from a wall.

2 Step your left foot forward into an open stance.

3 Extend your right arm to shoulder height, and rest the palm of your hand on the wall above you.

4 Keeping contact with the wall, allow your right arm to slowly circle back and down behind you, bringing your hand to rest just below shoulder height.

5 Open your chest and slightly bend your left knee, shifting your weight several inches forward.

6 Inhale and exhale deeply as you hold here for 15 to 30 seconds.

7 Switch sides and repeat three times on each arm.

TRICEP STRETCH

AFFECTED AREAS
Upper arms: *triceps, biceps*
Shoulders: *deltoids*

GOOD FOR
Counterbalance the downward pull of gravity on your arms by lifting your arms overhead and lengthening the sides of your body. You'll be able to loosen the area along the back of your arms as well as find some solace from tight shoulders.

LEVEL UP
Throw in a towel to ramp up this stretch. Grab one end of a rolled-up towel with your raised arm. Bring your opposite hand to your lower back and gently pull on the towel for 15 to 30 seconds.

REMEMBER
Try to engage your core muscles and open your chest as you perform this exercise. Keep your back straight throughout.

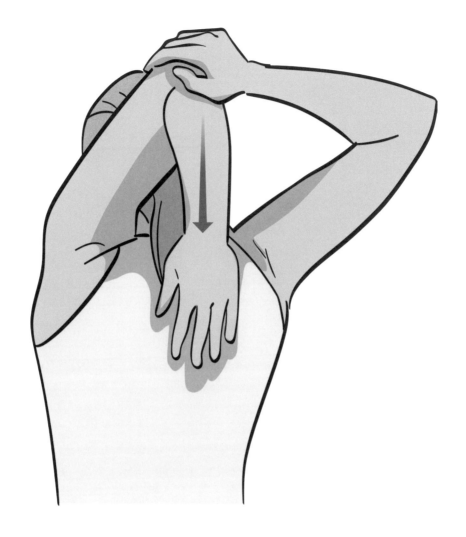

TYPE
STATIC

INSTRUCTIONS

1 Find a comfortable stance or a supported seated position.

2 Raise your left arm straight up along your left ear.

3 Turn your arm inward so that your palm is facing behind you.

4 Bring your right hand up to support your left elbow as you slowly bend your left elbow, reaching your palm to the back of your left shoulder.

5 Use your right hand to gently press your left elbow up and back for a stretch. Hold for 20 seconds at the top of the move and breathe.

6 Repeat three to four times.

WRIST FLEXION

AFFECTED AREAS

Upper arms: *biceps*

Forearms: *pronators, extensors, wrist flexors*

GOOD FOR

If your daily routine involves a lot of work with your hands or you have a hobby such as weight lifting, tennis, cooking, sewing, or gardening, this simple dynamic stretch will provide extensive relief through your wrists, forearms, and fingers.

LEVEL UP

Intensify the stretch by curling your extended fingers into a downward-facing fist. While keeping light pressure on the back of your wrist with your supporting hand, gently pull your fist down and away from your wrist.

REMEMBER

The shoulder of the extended arm will naturally want to lift, but try to keep both shoulders square and relaxed. Imagine pulling your shoulder blades down your back.

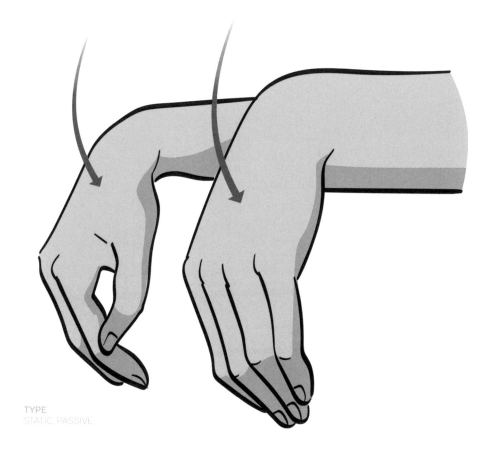

TYPE
STATIC, PASSIVE

INSTRUCTIONS

1   Begin either standing or seated, and extend your left arm straight out in front of you.

2   Press your left fingers and thumb together, and flex your wrist downward, pointing your fingers toward the floor.

3   With your right hand, gently press your left fingers bringing them closer in to your body.

4   Hold for 15 to 30 seconds, and repeat three to four times.

WRIST EXTENSION

AFFECTED AREAS

Forearms: *pronators, extensors, wrist flexors*

GOOD FOR

Your wrists and hands control and facilitate multiple daily tasks. Additionally, with the onset of texting, your hands rarely get a break for very long. Ease away painful wrist tension and hand cramping with this stretch—a little extension goes a long way.

LEVEL UP

For an additional challenge, hold your arm in place, and slowly bend and straighten your extended elbow while keeping light pressure on your palm with the supporting hand.

REMEMBER

It might surprise you how much stretch you feel with this simple move. You need only apply light pressure from your supporting hand to achieve a maximum stretch.

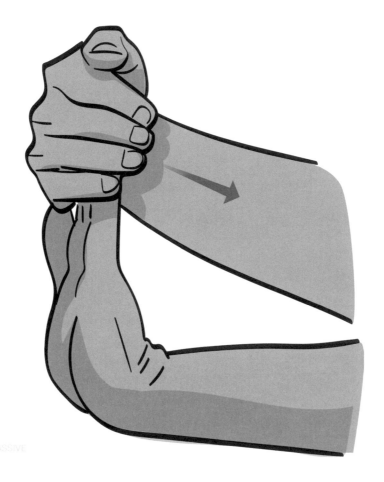

TYPE
STATIC, PASSIVE

INSTRUCTIONS

1   Begin seated or standing, and extend your right arm straight out in front of you, palm facing down.

2   Press your right fingers and thumb together, and pivot your wrist upward, pointing your fingers toward the ceiling.

3   Stretch from the base of your wrist as you bring your left hand to your right fingers.

4   With your left hand, gently press your right fingers back.

5   Hold for 15 to 30 seconds, and repeat three times on each wrist.

WALL-ASSISTED FOREARM STRETCH

AFFECTED AREAS

Upper arms: *biceps*

Forearms: *pronators, extensors, wrist flexors*

GOOD FOR

This highly effective stretch calls for you to turn your arm outward, exposing your inner forearm up to the ceiling while bringing your wrist into full extension. With the support of the wall, this stretch is ideal for anyone who needs a little extra help with balance.

LEVEL UP

Tilt your head away from the wall to feel more lengthening through your upper arm, shoulder, and neck.

REMEMBER

Try to open your fingers as wide as you can while your palm is in contact with the wall. This will assure an even stretch through your hand and fingers.

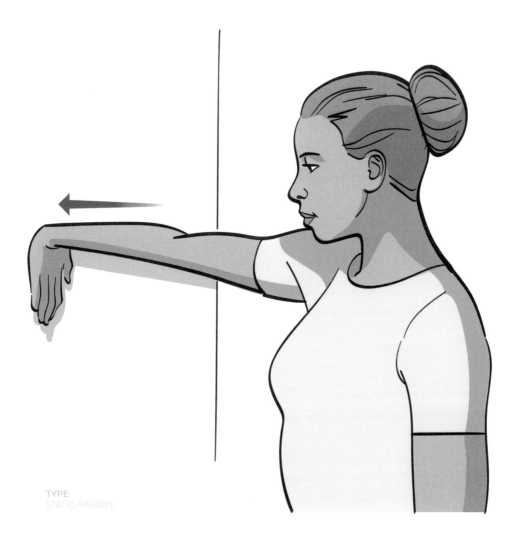

TYPE
STATIC, PASSIVE

INSTRUCTIONS

1   Stand with your right side positioned about arm's distance from a
    sturdy wall.
2   Bring your palm into contact with the wall, and spin your palm
    counterclockwise, pointing your fingers down toward the floor.
3   Press your palm into the wall by shifting your weight toward your arm.
4   Press your elbow up and open to the ceiling as you press your palm
    against the wall.
5   Hold for 15 to 20 seconds, and repeat on the opposite arm.
6   Perform three sets.

PRAYER HANDS

AFFECTED AREAS

Forearms: *flexors, pronators, extensors*

Wrists

GOOD FOR

Achieving the symmetry of this pose calls for you to focus on the midline of your body as you press your hands together and open the front of your chest. Prayer hands may help alleviate pain associated with ailments such as tennis elbow and arthritis.

LEVEL UP

When you're ready, advance to this dynamic variation. As you stretch through your arms, slowly extend your prayer hands above your head, keeping your palms pressed together, and slowly lower your hands back down toward the center of your chest. Repeat for up to 60 seconds.

REMEMBER

To achieve the ultimate symmetry of this stretch, be sure to form a straight line from elbow to elbow and along your forearms while keeping your palms pressed together.

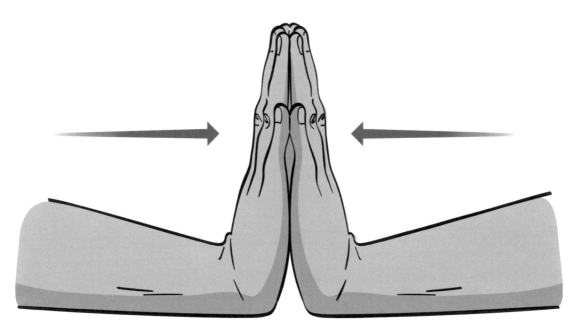

TYPE
STATIC, ACTIVE

INSTRUCTIONS

1   Begin in a comfortable position either standing or sitting.

2   Inhale and press your palms together in front of your chest, with your
    fingers touching your chin.

3   Exhale as you press the base of your palms, fingers, and thumbs firmly
    together and lower your hands toward your waist.

4   Hold for 15 to 30 seconds, and repeat three times.

PRAYER HANDS FLEXION

AFFECTED AREAS
Forearms: *flexors, pronators, extensors*

GOOD FOR
Your wrists are each made up of eight small bones. Connecting into your wrists and hands are multiple muscles and tendons of your forearms that help control your hand movements. This flexing stretch is wonderful for loosening up the muscles in your forearms, wrists, and hands.

LEVEL UP
For an added challenge, try moving your hands and fingers from left to right while pressing the tops of your hands together.

REMEMBER
You need not try right away to reach a full range of wrist movement in this stretch. Trust your limits and work within them; eventually, a wider range will come to you through practice.

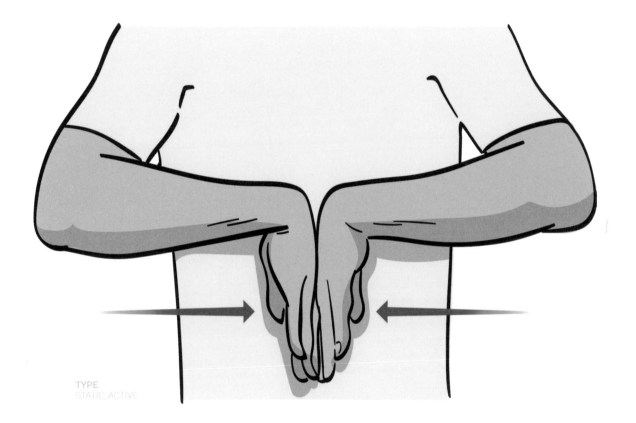

INSTRUCTIONS

1   Begin in a comfortable position either standing or sitting.

2   Inhale and press the tops of your hands together in front of your chest into an inverted Prayer Hands position.

3   Exhale as you focus on keeping contact between the tops of your hands and fingers and lowering your shoulders and elbows.

4   Hold for 10 to 15 seconds.

FINGER STRETCH

AFFECTED AREAS

Forearms: *flexors, pronators, wrist extensors*

Hands

Fingers

GOOD FOR

Hours of scrolling on your computer or texting on your phone can lead to overuse of your fingers, causing stiffness, tenderness, and pain in your arms, elbows, and wrists. Take some time to open up the spaces between your fingers with this simple stretch.

LEVEL UP

For an added stretch through your wrists, flip your hands over so that your palms are facing up. Now, curl your fingers into tight fists and hold for 10 seconds. Then slowly release your fists and open your hands. Wiggle your fingers and repeat three times.

REMEMBER

Your thumbs can easily become more immobile than your fingers, so pay attention to how you splay your hands open. Give extra attention to your thumbs, pulling them gently open and in toward each other.

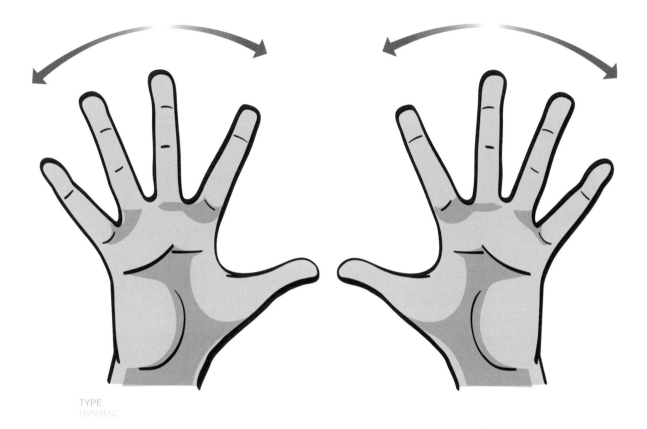

TYPE
DYNAMIC

INSTRUCTIONS

1   Choose a comfortable place where you can stand easily or can sit with support from a chair.
2   Extend your arms out in front of your chest, keeping your elbows slightly bent.
3   Press your fingers and thumbs together so that there's no space between them, and hold for five seconds.
4   Next splay your fingers wide open, creating a lot of space between them. Hold for five seconds.
5   Repeat five times.

FIST ROTATION

AFFECTED AREAS

Forearms: *flexors, pronators, extensors*
Neck

GOOD FOR

Try these deceivingly simple fist rotations at your own leisure. You may discover that your range of motion differs between hands. Enjoy some relief through your neck and arms as an important reminder of the interconnectedness that exists throughout your body.

LEVEL UP

For a more intense stretch through your wrists and forearms, hold a small weighted ball in each hand and wrap your fingers evenly around them. Perform your wrist circles in each direction.

REMEMBER

The focus of this exercise is to independently isolate the movement of your wrists from the movement of your forearms. Pay attention to when you want to move your forearms and when you are able to fully isolate your wrists: This will reveal where your hands are tightest.

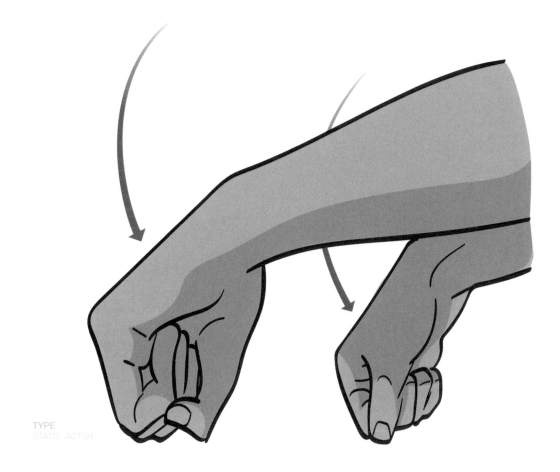

TYPE
STATIC, ACTIVE

INSTRUCTIONS

1   Loosely extend your arms out in front of your body.

2   Turn your palms down, and curl in your fingers to make soft fists.

3   Slowly begin to make isolated circular movements with your fists,
    keeping your forearms steady.

4   Perform five rotations in one direction, then reverse the direction for
    another five rotations.

5   Do three sets on each wrist.

THUMB STRETCH

AFFECTED AREAS

Thumbs: *flexors, extensors, pro nadirs*

GOOD FOR

Our hands get a workout all day long: We text, type, play musical instruments, and do various chores. Yet rarely do we take the time to pamper our tired hands and, in particular, our thumbs. These isolated stretches are most impactful when you're fully relaxed.

LEVEL UP

Turn this stretch into a dynamic exercise and rotate your thumb in circles with your opposite hand. Keep your palm steady as you move your thumb.

ON THE FLY

This is a very soothing stretch that can be done seated, lying down, or standing. It is especially valuable because you can perform it anywhere you go.

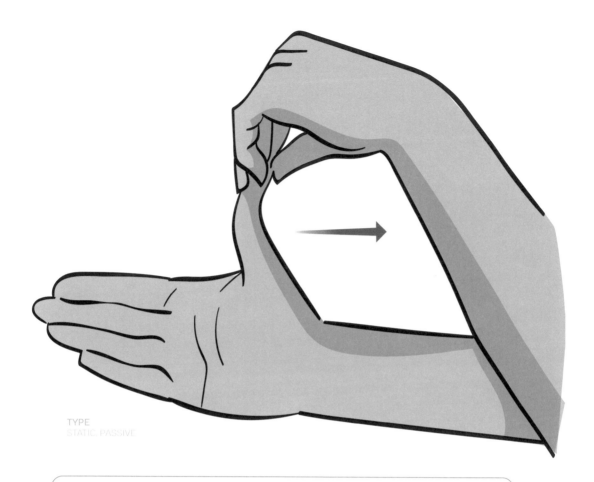

INSTRUCTIONS

1 Find a comfortable place to sit.

2 Hold your right hand in front of your chest, with your palm facing your chest.

3 Wrap your left hand around your right thumb. Keeping your right hand in line with your forearm, push your thumb downward, and hold for 10 seconds.

4 Flex your wrist toward your chest. Push your thumb toward your forearm, and hold for 10 seconds.

5 Next, extend your wrist so your palm is perpendicular to your chest. Again push on your thumb, and hold for 10 seconds.

6 Repeat on the opposite hand.

CHAPTER
8

CORE & HIPS

Core stretches benefit a group of critical muscles, toning your abdominals along the front and sides of your torso. These stretches improve your balance and sports performance. Hip stretches are also essential for maintaining proper balance and coordination. By performing core and hip stretches regularly, you'll improve the range of motion in your lower body and help protect against injuries.

HIP TWIST

AFFECTED AREAS

Buttocks: *gluteals*

Hip rotators: *piriformis, quadratus femoris*

Abdomen: *abdominal obliques, transverse abdominus*

GOOD FOR

Open those hard-to-reach muscles that wrap across your lower back and hips, and along the sides of your torso. The twisting movement of this stretch helps improve posture and lower-back pain.

LEVEL UP

Intensify this twisted movement by pushing down strongly into your right hand. Lift your core up and in, and straighten your left arm, reaching your left fingertips down to the floor.

ON THE FLY

If you find it challenging to sit up straight through your lower spine in this pose, place a rolled-up towel, yoga block, or firm pillow under your hips for support.

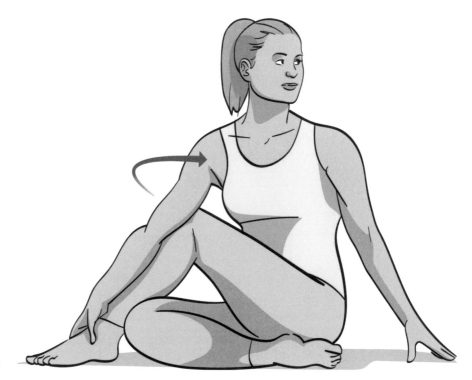

INSTRUCTIONS

1   Sit with your legs extended in front of you.

2   Step your left foot over your right knee, and rest your left foot on the floor just outside your right knee.

3   Place your left hand on the floor near your left hip, and put weight on it for support.

4   Raise your right arm, pull in your abs, and root your left foot down. Lengthen through your spine as you twist your torso to your left.

5   Lower your right arm. Bend your right elbow, and place it on the outside of your left knee.

6   Push down into your left arm and twist your upper torso, turning your head to look to your left.

7   Hold for 20 to 30 seconds, and repeat three times on each side.

COBRA

AFFECTED AREAS

Abdomen: *rectus abdominus, abdominal obliques*

Chest: *pectorals*

Back: *erector spinae*

Hip flexors: *psoas*

GOOD FOR

A sedentary lifestyle can be detrimental to the health of your hips and core, weakening the muscles that support your upper and lower body. Try the Cobra to alleviate tightness in the front of your hips and to counteract slouching and a tucked-in pelvis.

LEVEL UP

Once you're confident with the basic Cobra, intensify the stretch. Begin in the same position except bring your hands slightly farther down from your shoulders toward your chest. Push into your hands, and lift your body up a little higher.

REMEMBER

To protect your lower back during this upward movement, be sure to activate your lower abdominals. Before you push down into your hands to lift up your body, squeeze in those abs and keep them tight.

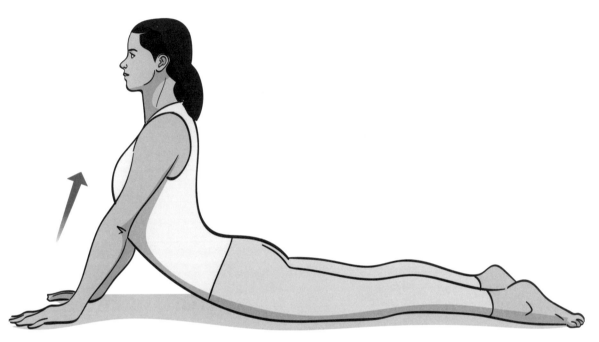

TYPE
STATIC ACTIVE

INSTRUCTIONS

1   Lie facedown on the floor with your legs extended straight behind you and your feet about shoulder-width apart.

2   Press your forearms into the floor at the sides of your head.

3   Strongly pull in your core, and push down into your hands as you slowly lift your upper body from the floor. Rise up only as far as is comfortable.

4   Roll your shoulders back and try to straighten your arms.

5   Point your toes and keep the tops of your feet in contact with the floor.

6   Lift your chin, open your chest, and gaze slightly upward

7   Hold for 20 to 30 seconds and breathe deeply. Repeat three times.

BUTTERFLY

AFFECTED AREAS

Inner thighs: *adductors*

Hips: *abductors*

Buttocks: *gluteals*

GOOD FOR

The Butterfly is a great hip flexor stretch for everyone, from athletes to office workers. Allow gravity to assist you in opening your hips and inner thighs as you lower your knees out to your sides. By keeping your hips limber, you'll also help protect against groin injuries.

LEVEL UP

When you're ready for more of a challenge, pull in your feet closer to your groin and hold your ankles. Push gently on your legs with your forearms to lower your knees farther toward the floor, and bow your head toward your feet.

REMEMBER

If your hips are very tight or you are struggling to sit on the floor with a straight back, add some support by tucking a folded towel or a small yoga block under your hips.

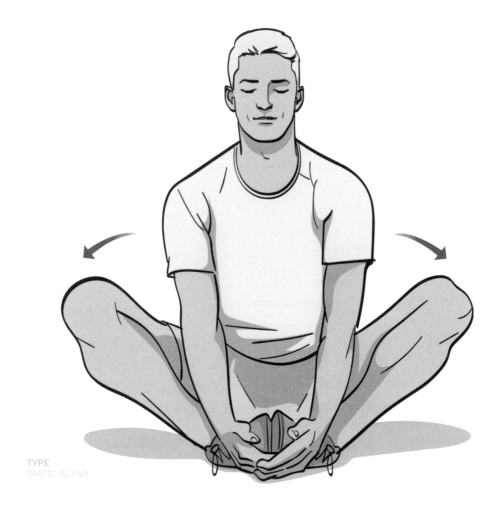

INSTRUCTIONS

1 Take a moment to find a comfortable place to sit on a firm surface. Extend your legs out in front of you, and support your body by placing your hands at the sides of your hips.

2 Bend your knees, turning your legs outward.

3 Reach forward, place your hands on your ankles, and press the soles of your feet together.

4 Pull in your abdominals and lengthen through your lower back. Allow your knees to drop open and down with the pull of gravity.

5 Breathe deeply and hold for 20 to 30 seconds.

6 Repeat three times.

PIRIFORMIS STRETCH

AFFECTED AREAS

Buttocks: *piriformis, gluteals*
Thighs: *hamstrings*
Lower back: *erector spinae*

GOOD FOR

Your lower back and hips are sensitive areas that can easily become tight and lose their mobility. If you are prone to stiff hips or sciatic pain, this stretch may alleviate some of your discomfort. When performed regularly, this excellent exercise can yield long-lasting results.

LEVEL UP

Add an exercise band to this stretch to help isolate the targeted muscles. Wrap a short exercise band around the ankle of the supporting leg. Allow the knee of that leg to tip outward, and gently pull on your ankle for a deep stretch.

REMEMBER

Keep your spine long and connected to the floor during this stretch. This essential exercise can be done on the fly, as long as you have the floor space to perform it.

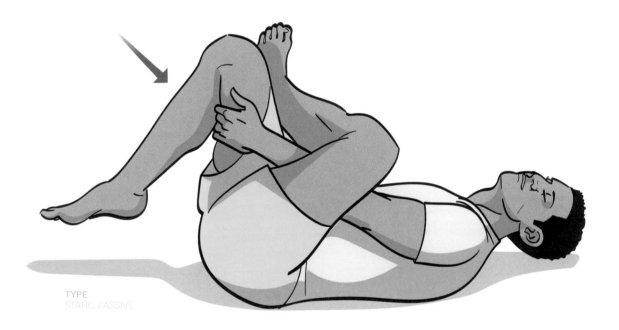

INSTRUCTIONS

1   Lie down on a comfortable but firm surface. Bend your knees, keeping the soles of your feet on the floor.

2   Cross your right ankle over your left thigh, and rest your right shin on your left leg.

3   Reach behind your left thigh, and if you can, clasp your hands together. Gently pull your left leg in toward your chest, allowing your left foot to lift from the floor.

4   Breathe deeply and hold for 20 to 30 seconds. Repeat on the opposite side.

5   Perform three sets.

SIDE STRETCH

AFFECTED AREAS

Abdomen: *abdominal obliques, transverse abdominus*
Back: *latissimus dorsi*
Buttocks: *piriformis*
Inner thighs: *adductors*

GOOD FOR

Sometimes you need to rebalance your vertical posture by stretching horizontally. If you've spent a good deal of time standing or sitting with your spine positioned vertically, give yourself a deep opening through the sides of your torso, hips, and hamstrings with this horizontal stretch.

LEVEL UP

Wrap a resistance band around the foot of your extended leg, and hold the ends with your overhead hand. Pull gently on the band to increase the stretch along your side.

REMEMBER

If this is a new move for you, take your time positioning yourself. Ideally, you should work toward bringing your torso closer and closer to your extended leg.

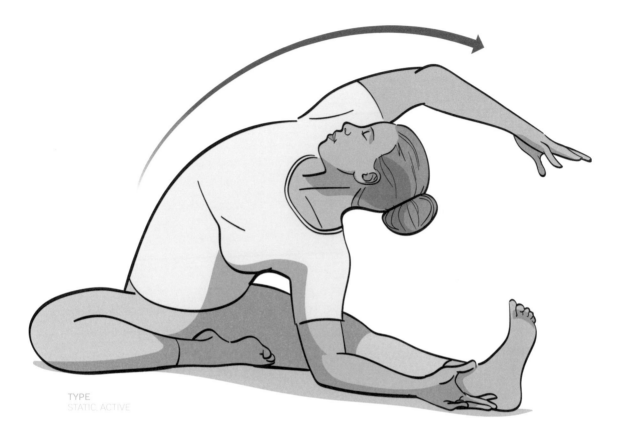

TYPE
STATIC, ACTIVE

INSTRUCTIONS

1   Sit on the floor and open your legs out to your sides as far as you are comfortable.

2   Bend your left knee and place the outside of your left foot on the floor in front of your pelvis.

3   Extend your left arm up, engage your core, and reach your left hand up and over toward your right side.

4   Allow your right hand to slide along the floor in front of your right leg down to your ankle.

5   Gaze between your arms and breathe deeply as you hold for 20 to 30 seconds.

6   Repeat three times on each side.

CENTER SPLIT

AFFECTED AREAS
Inner thighs: *adductors*
Back: *erector spinae*

GOOD FOR
The splits! As soon as we hear the word *split*, many of us cringe or assume it's impossible to achieve. Actually, performing a split, like all stretches, is something you can work toward gradually. It's an excellent hip opener to improve the mobility in your lower body.

LEVEL UP
Once you've reached a point of relaxation in your split, inhale and gently roll your hips forward while rotating your legs outward in opposition to your hips. As you progress, little by little, you may even be able to touch your chest to the floor in front of you.

REMEMBER
Go for this center split only when you are thoroughly warmed up and at your most limber throughout lower back, legs, and your hips. The split is best performed at the very end of your stretching routine.

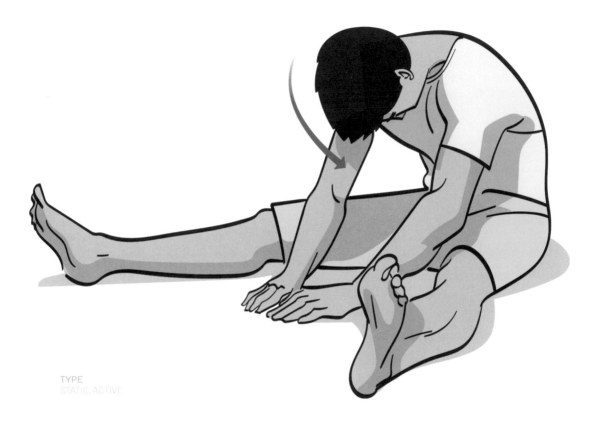

INSTRUCTIONS

1   Sit on the floor and open your legs wide. If you need more support through your lower back, place a pillow or folded towel under your hips.

2   Place your palms on the floor in front of you.

3   Pull up through your core and in toward your lower spine, and slowly walk your hands forward away from your hips.

4   Pause when you've reached your maximum stretch.

5   Inhale and exhale deeply for up to 30 seconds.

6   Repeat twice.

TRIANGLE POSE

AFFECTED AREAS

Abdomen: *abdominal obliques, transverse abdominus*

Back: *erector spinae*

Inner thighs: *adductors*

GOOD FOR

With its origins in yoga, the Triangle Pose offers a deep stretch along the back and front of your lower abdomen while lengthening the sides of your torso and back. This is a fantastic stretch if you're experiencing stiffness through your lower back and hips.

LEVEL UP

For an advanced stretch, lower your hand from your ankle down to the floor in front of your foot, and try to place your palm on the floor. Push forward with your pelvis and lengthen through your arms, forming a straight line from hand to hand.

REMEMBER

If this stretch is too challenging for you at first, you may place your hand on your shin rather than your ankle. Find what works for your body and gradually intensify the stretch.

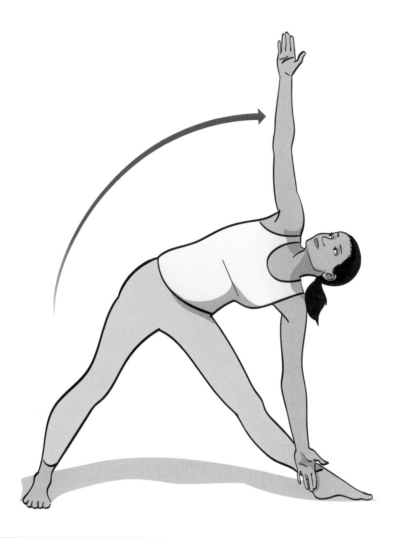

TYPE
STATIC, ACTIVE

INSTRUCTIONS

1 Stand tall and face forward. Step your legs in a wide stance of about four feet apart.

2 Turn your left toes out to the side and keep your right foot facing forward.

3 Open your arms out to your sides and shift your hips slightly to the right, bending at the waist.

4 Slide your left fingers down to your left ankle, and extend your right arm up toward the ceiling.

5 Look up toward your right hand and hold for 20 to 30 seconds.

6 Repeat on the opposite side. Perform three sets.

SEATED SPINAL TWIST

AFFECTED AREAS

Abdomen: *abdominal obliques, transverse abdominus*
Hips: *adductors*
Buttocks: *piriformis, gluteals*

GOOD FOR

A gentle turn of your spine in one direction, with support from your hands, is an easy way to give yourself a relaxing and passive stretch along your lower back, hips, and torso. This one is good for all ages and body types.

LEVEL UP

To challenge your balance, sit on a large fitness ball with your feet flat on the floor and about hip-width apart. As you move into your twist, press down through your feet into the floor and pull your core upward and inward.

REMEMBER

With cross-legged stretches, it's always good to alternate the upper and lower legs. This gives you an even balance throughout the body and a chance to work the nondominant body parts.

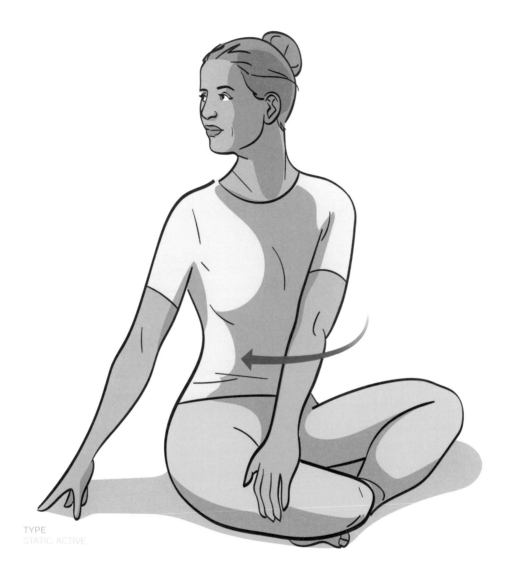

TYPE
STATIC, ACTIVE

INSTRUCTIONS

1 Take a seat on the floor or in a sturdy chair and loosely cross your legs.
2 Keeping your back upright, begin twisting your body to the right.
3 Reach your left arm across your chest to touch your right knee, and reach your right arm behind your right hip.
4 Turn your head to look over your right shoulder and hold for 30 seconds.
5 Repeat three times to each side.

SIDE LUNGE

AFFECTED AREAS

Thighs: *quadriceps, hamstrings, adductors*
Buttocks: *gluteals, piriformis*

GOOD FOR

By shifting your weight to one hip and holding this lunge, you are activating the larger muscle groups that support your pelvis and hips while strengthening the smaller muscle groups. This isometric stretch may help mitigate lower-back pain and hip stiffness stemming from muscle weakness.

LEVEL UP

To advance this move, add a little weight. Hold a small weighted ball or dumbbell with both hands and raise it in front of your chest as you lunge to the side.

REMEMBER

It is important to maintain good form in this move. To protect your knee joint from overstretching, be sure that your bent knee does not extend farther to the side than your ankle. If necessary, step your feet wider apart to achieve this alignment.

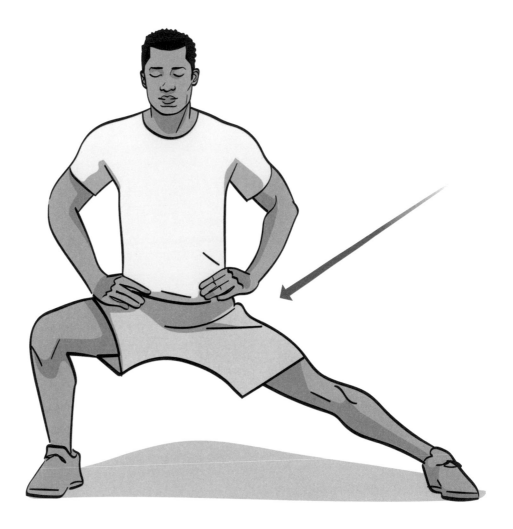

TYPE
STATIC, ACTIVE

INSTRUCTIONS

1   Begin by standing up straight. Step your legs open as wide as you can,
    and turn both feet slightly outward.

2   Place your hands on your hips and pull in your core muscles.

3   Slowly bend your right knee, keeping your back straight.

4   Take several deep breaths, holding the stretch for up to 30 seconds.

5   Repeat on the opposite side and perform three sets.

PIGEON

AFFECTED AREAS

Buttocks: *piriformis, gluteals*
Thighs: *adductors, hamstrings*
Back: *erector spinae, quadratus lumborum*

GOOD FOR

If you develop pain in the muscles that wrap along the sides of your pelvis, you may also be losing muscle strength and mobility. Settle into the Pigeon pose and enjoy a deep opening around your hip joints and through the surrounding supporting muscles.

LEVEL UP

Advance this yoga-based stretch by keeping your torso upright. Rest your palms outside of your hips and press your fingertips into the floor.

REMEMBER

Keep some weight in your hands so they can support your body weight and add to the range of your stretch.

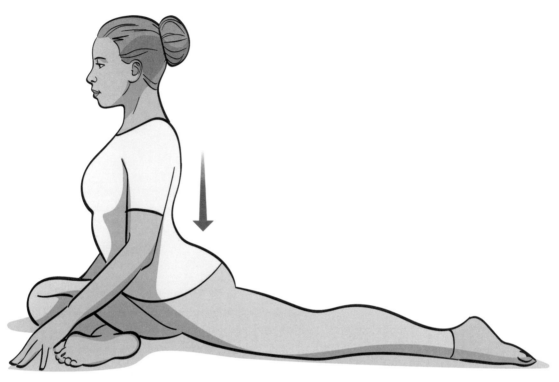

TYPE
STATIC, ACTIVE

INSTRUCTIONS

1   Begin on all fours with your hands and knees on the floor.

2   Pressing your weight into your hands, shift your right knee across your body and rest it on the floor in front of you. Your knee should be in line with the center of your chest.

3   Extend your left leg behind you, keeping it bent, as you slowly walk your hands forward.

4   Rest your elbows on the floor and clasp your hands, turning your gaze forward.

5   Hold for 20 to 30 seconds and repeat twice on each side.

HIP FLEXOR STRETCH

AFFECTED AREAS

Hip flexors: *psoas, iliacus, sartorius*
Thighs: *quadriceps, hamstrings, adductors*

GOOD FOR

This stretch reaches deep into your hips and opens the muscles around the front and back of your pelvis, while lengthening your core. Because this stretch requires a deep folding in your hips, you should be thoroughly warmed up in your back, hips, and legs.

LEVEL UP

Give yourself a deeper stretch by keeping both legs straight. Begin standing and step your left foot far forward. Lean your torso forward, and lower your hands to floor on either side of your left foot. Flex your left foot and hold for up to 30 seconds.

REMEMBER

Be sure to keep your hips square rather than shifted to one side. Relax your neck and shoulders as you lean forward.

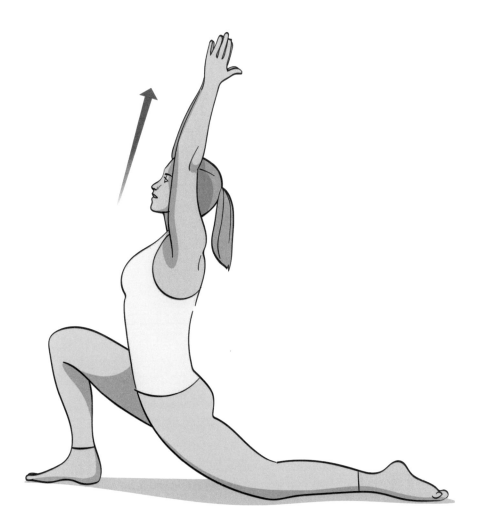

TYPE
STATIC, ACTIVE

INSTRUCTIONS

1   Begin by kneeling on the floor with the tops of your feet touching the floor.

2   Extend your left leg forward and place your left foot on the floor, keeping a slight bend in your knee.

3   Raise your arms overhead, keeping your back straight, and find your balance.

4   Next, flex your extended left foot and lean your torso forward. Lower your hands to the floor at your sides for balance.

5   Hold for 20 seconds and repeat on the opposite side.

6   Perform three sets.

ALTERNATE HIP INTERNAL ROTATION

AFFECTED AREAS

Buttocks: *piriformis, gluteus minimus*
Thighs: *adductors, abductors*
Lower back: *psoas, erector spinae*

GOOD FOR

Internally rotating the hips is a great way to counterbalance all the outward hip movements that we perform daily such as walking, sitting, and standing. This stretch improves flexibility through your hips and pelvis while opening the hard-to-reach areas of your lower back.

LEVEL UP

With your legs wide and feet flat on the floor, let both knees drop together to your right side in a controlled manner. Return to the starting position and lower your legs to your left. Perform 10 repetitions.

REMEMBER

Engage your abs the entire time. Breathe deeply as you perform this movement slowly and deliberately.

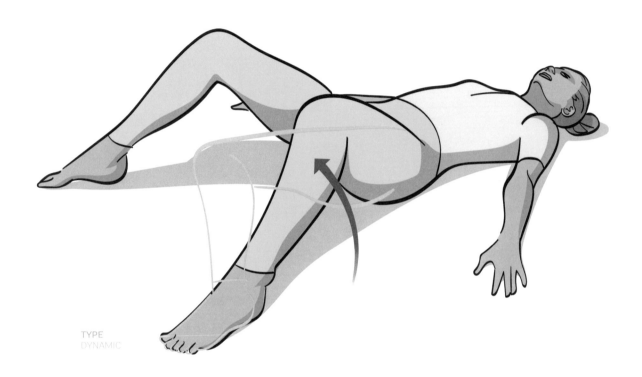

TYPE
DYNAMIC

INSTRUCTIONS

1   Lie on your back with your knees bent at about 90 degrees and your
    feet shoulder-width apart.

2   Extend your arms out to your sides, and press your palms into the floor.

3   Slowly lower your left knee toward the floor, allowing your left foot to
    rotate inward, and return to the starting position.

4   Lower your right knee and return to the starting position.

5   Repeat 10 times on each side.

LEGS, KNEES, FEET & ANKLES

Your legs are the foundation of your body, supplying support and stability. Toned, flexible muscles in your thighs, knees, calves, ankles, and feet can minimize aches and pains, improve posture, help prevent injuries, and speed recovery time after engaging in sports or workouts.

TOE TOUCH STANDING

AFFECTED AREAS
Thighs: *hamstrings*
Calves: *gastrocnemius, soleus*
Buttocks: *glutes*

GOOD FOR
Moving through this Toe Touch stretch is a great way to feel the connection of muscles from your hips, along the backs of your legs, and down to your feet. The inversion also helps get your blood flowing.

LEVEL UP
Hold a weighted ball in your hands to begin. As you bend forward, lower the ball toward your toes, allowing gravity to deepen the stretch along the backs of your legs.

ON THE FLY
This stretch is great for anytime you feel tightness in the back of your legs. Find a comfortable location that allows you enough space to reach for your toes, and go for it.

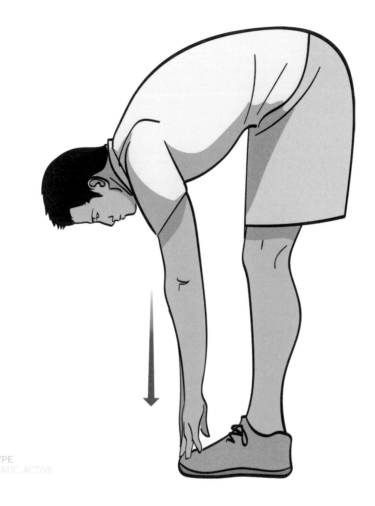

TYPE
STATIC, ACTIVE

INSTRUCTIONS

1   Stand up straight, lengthening your spine, and place your feet shoulder-width apart.

2   Lower your head and slowly curl your torso forward, one vertebra at a time, bending from your hips. Allow your arms to dangle loosely beneath you.

3   If you can, touch your toes, and breathe deeply, inhaling and exhaling.

4   Hold for 10 seconds.

5   Roll up slowly through your lower back and spine, and return to neutral position.

6   Repeat three to five times.

STANDING QUADRICEP STRETCH

AFFECTED AREAS
Thighs: quadriceps
Shins: *tibialis*

GOOD FOR
If you've ever been sitting for so long that when you stand up, the front of your hips feel stuck and cramped, this stretch may be beneficial for you. Release tension and stiffness from sedentary postures with this standing quadricep stretch.

LEVEL UP
For a stretch along your outer thigh and iliotibial band, grab your raised foot with the opposite hand. Allow your raised leg to turn out slightly, and bring your heel across to the opposite hip.

REMEMBER
Press your pelvis forward, and keep your hips flat to the front without arching your lower spine. If needed, use a wall or a chair for balance.

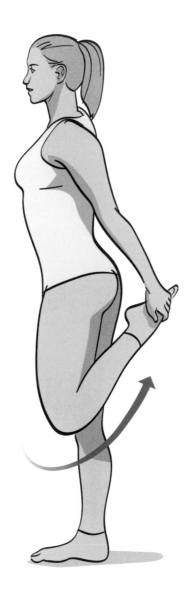

TYPE
STATIC, PASSIVE

INSTRUCTIONS

1   Stand straight with your feet together and engage your abs.
2   Bend your left knee, bringing your left foot up behind you.
3   Reach your left arm behind you, and wrap your hand around the top of your left foot. Bring your right hand onto your right hip to help with balance or let it hang at your side.
4   Pull your left heel in toward your left hip and hold for 10 to 15 seconds
5   Return to neutral position, and repeat two to three times on each leg.

HAMSTRING STRETCH

AFFECTED AREAS

Thighs: *hamstrings, quadriceps*

Calves: *gastrocnemius, soleus*

GOOD FOR

Utilizing the pull of gravity to stretch your leg makes this simple Hamstring Stretch great for all ages and body types. This move is good for warming up before a workout, cooling down after a run, or searching for relief from lower-back pain.

LEVEL UP

Use a resistance band or rolled-up towel to maximize your range in this stretch. Wrap the band under your raised foot, and hold the ends with both hands. As you straighten your leg, use the band to pull your leg in closer toward your chest.

REMEMBER

If you have very tight hamstrings, it may cause you to hike up your shoulders and tense the surrounding neck muscles. Remember to press the back of your neck flat against the floor and gently press your shoulders down and away from your ears.

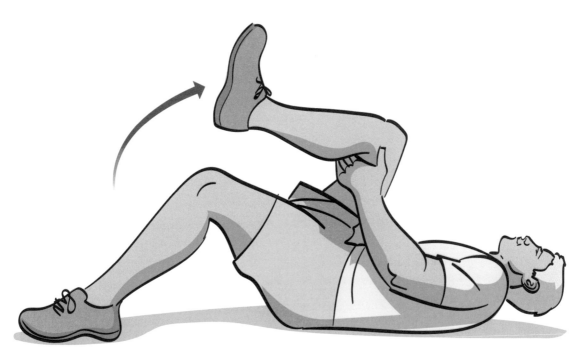

INSTRUCTIONS

1 Lie on your back with your knees bent. Place both feet flat on the floor.

2 Lift your left leg into the air, and wrap your hands behind your leg just above your knee.

3 Engage your abs, flex your left foot, and slowly straighten your knee.

4 Hold here for 15 to 20 seconds, and return to neutral position.

5 Repeat three to five times on each leg.

FOOT SICKLE

AFFECTED AREAS
Shins: *tibialis anterior*
Feet: *extensors*
Toes

GOOD FOR

Many of us spend hours on our feet daily and don't give them enough attention. Pain in your hips, knees, and lower back is sometimes related to how you stand on your feet. Try this isolated Foot Sickle stretch to rejuvenate your outer shins and ankles.

LEVEL UP

To get a deeper stretch through your ankle joint, hold your foot just below your toes. Pull the middle of your foot up toward you while keeping the support of the other hand on your shin.

REMEMBER

This stretch can be done either seated in a chair or with support of the floor. Take it wherever you go. Just remember to take off your shoes first so you can isolate the stretch accordingly.

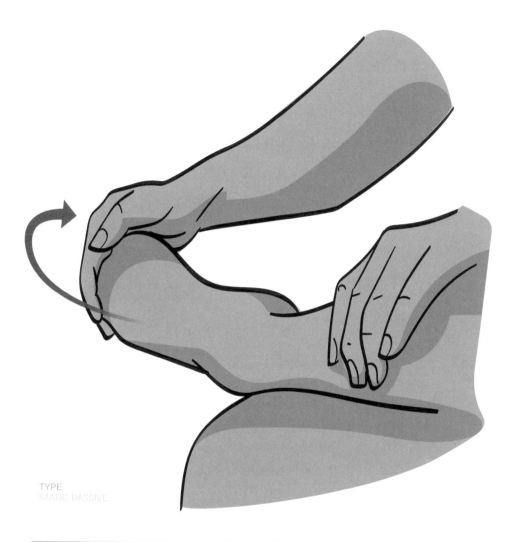

TYPE
STATIC, PASSIVE

INSTRUCTIONS

1   Find a comfortable seated position, and bring your right foot up to cross over your left knee.

2   Support your right shin with your right hand while you wrap your left hand around your right toes.

3   Isolating your toes and foot, pull your right toes toward your left shoulder.

4   Hold for 10 to 15 seconds and repeat on the opposite foot.

5   Perform three sets.

TOE STRETCH

AFFECTED AREAS

Feet: *extensors*

Arches of feet: *plantar fascia*

Toes

GOOD FOR

Your range of motion may vary significantly from toe to toe as you try out these easy Toe Stretch isolations. In addition to targeting your toes, this stretch series soothes tired ankles and arches. It's perfect for general foot pain and for cooling down overworked feet.

LEVEL UP

When stretching your toes, try moving them in a new direction. Instead of tugging them apart, push them up and down, working each neighboring toe against the other.

REMEMBER

Even though your toes are small, they play an important part in carrying and dispersing the weight of your body. Remember to care for them and be gentle when stretching.

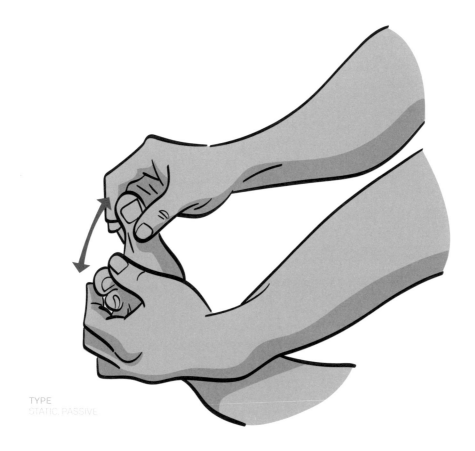

INSTRUCTIONS

1   Find a comfortable seated position, and cross your right ankle over your left knee.
2   Begin by pulling your big toe away from your second toe.
3   Next, tug apart your second toe and middle toes.
4   Continue separating your toes this way down to your pinky toe.
5   Breathe deeply as you stretch, and repeat three to five times on each foot.

HIGH KNEE WALKING

AFFECTED AREAS
Thighs: *quadriceps, hamstrings*
Buttocks: *gluteals*

GOOD FOR

This high knee stretch has many benefits. Not only are you stretching through your knees and upper legs, you're also improving strength, coordination, and circulation in your core, exterior leg muscles, and hip joints. This dynamic stretch is ideal for warming up before a run.

LEVEL UP

For an added challenge, strap on some light ankle weights and proceed slowly. This will serve to strengthen your quadriceps as well as improve your balance. Perform five repetitions on each leg.

REMEMBER

This is a simple exercise that you can do anywhere. It is especially useful as a warm-up before various sports and aerobic workouts. Engage your core to help you keep the movement fluid and controlled.

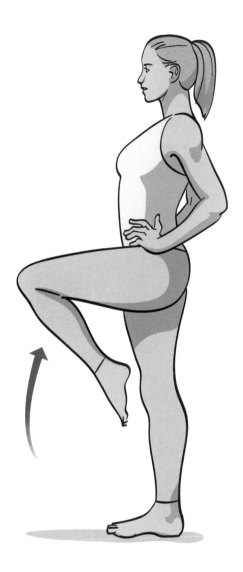

TYPE
DYNAMIC

INSTRUCTIONS

1 Begin by standing straight with your feet hip-width apart. Place your hands on your hips.

2 Shift your weight onto your left foot, engage your core, and bring your left knee up high so that your hamstrings are parallel to the floor.

3 Lower your foot to the floor, stepping forward, and repeat with the opposite leg.

4 Continue walking for 10 repetitions on each leg.

5 Turn around and repeat three times.

ANKLE CIRCLES

AFFECTED AREAS
Shins: *tibialis anterior*
Arches of feet: *plantar fascia*
Toes

GOOD FOR
When you move your body parts in a circular manner, you help promote circulation, mobility, and relaxation. Here, by isolating your ankle joint and moving it in a smooth circular motion through its maximum range, you can relax your tired, achy feet and enhance their flexibility.

LEVEL UP
Increase the range of motion by using your hand to assist your ankle through a wider circle. Place your left leg on your right thigh, and press your right palm against the sole of your left foot. Hold the sides of your arch and gently rotate your ankle in each direction.

REMEMBER
This stretch can be done just about anywhere, with or without your shoes on. If your feet are feeling achy or swollen, find a wall to help with your balance and circle your ankles a few times in each direction.

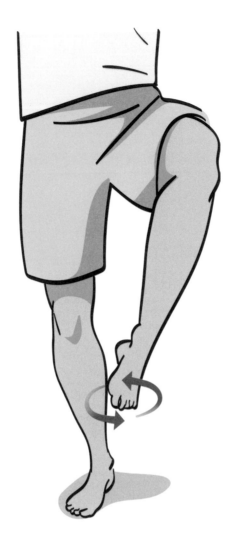

TYPE
DYNAMIC

INSTRUCTIONS

1   Stand straight with your feet hip-width apart, and place your hands on your hips.

2   Bend your right knee, and lift your right foot up from the floor.

3   Trace a small circle counterclockwise with your right foot by pointing your toes down to the floor, out to your right, up to the ceiling, and in toward your left leg.

4   Perform five circles, then reverse the direction, tracing a circle clockwise.

5   Repeat five times on each foot.

POINTE & FLEX

AFFECTED AREAS

Shins: *tibialis anterior*

Calves: *gastrocnemius, soleus*

Arches of feet: *plantar fascia*

Toes

GOOD FOR

Unless you are a ballerina and are always on your toes, your feet are probably in a flexed position most of the day. Try this stretch to invigorate tired feet and loosen up the tightness in the stiff joints of your lower leg with this point-and-flex movement.

LEVEL UP

Wrap a resistance band or rolled-up towel behind the soles of your feet. Pull firmly on the band as you flex your feet. Push the backs of your legs into the floor, and push away with your heels as you curl your toes back toward your shins.

REMEMBER

When you're able to take a break from your daily routine, find a quiet location to sit either on the floor or in a chair, slip off your shoes, and work your feet through this pointe stretch.

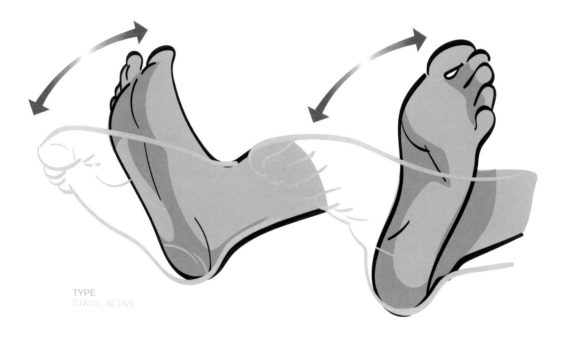

TYPE
STATIC, ACTIVE

INSTRUCTIONS

1 Sit comfortably and extend your legs straight in front of you.

2 Curl your feet and toes away from your shins and toward the floor, bringing each foot into a full pointe.

3 Hold for 15 seconds and return to neutral position.

4 Now flex your feet by engaging your calves and pushing out through your heels while pulling your toes back toward you.

5 Hold for 10 seconds and return to neutral.

6 Repeat three to five times.

TIBIALIS KNEE STRETCH

AFFECTED AREAS

Shins: *tibialis anterior*

Calves: *gastrocnemius, soleus*

GOOD FOR

Utilizing the force of gravity, this move allows you to root down through your hips and lengthen your shins, calves, and feet. This restorative stretch relieves stiffness through your legs and feet. It may also help decrease calf and ankle swelling after air travel.

LEVEL UP

When you're ready for a much more advanced version of this stretch, try the yoga-based Reclining Hero Pose. Kneel with your feet wider than hip-width apart, and place your arms behind you. Slowly lower your back toward the floor.

REMEMBER

If you have knee pain and are not able to kneel comfortably in the basic pose, tuck a folded blanket or towel under your hips for extra support.

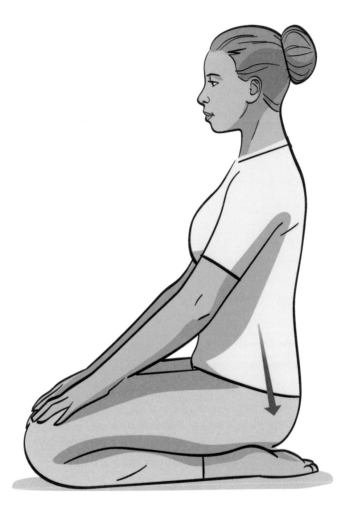

TYPE
PASSIVE

INSTRUCTIONS

1 Begin by kneeling on all fours on a solid surface with the tops of your feet on the floor.

2 Slowly bring your legs together so that they touch.

3 Gradually tip your hips back toward your feet and come into a full kneel, bringing your hips to your heels.

4 Engage your abs and sit up straight. Rest your hands on your thighs and breathe deeply.

5 Hold for 30 seconds and repeat three times.

SUMO SQUAT

AFFECTED AREAS
Thighs: *quadriceps, hamstrings, abductors, adductors*

GOOD FOR
Take a wide-open stance and come into the Sumo stretch to activate and lengthen muscles deep in your hips and legs. You'll also build stamina and strength through your core. Holding the correct sumo position is challenging—you need to bend your knees deeply all while keeping your abs in and up. This is a great stretch to do before working out, running, or playing sports.

LEVEL UP
Challenge the strength in your core and in your legs by holding a weighted medicine ball or kettle bell overhead as you bend your knees and slowly lower into your sumo position.

REMEMBER
This move can be performed anywhere, assuming your clothing allows for it. Find a space wide enough for your squat position and be sure to keep your core and back muscles engaged the whole time.

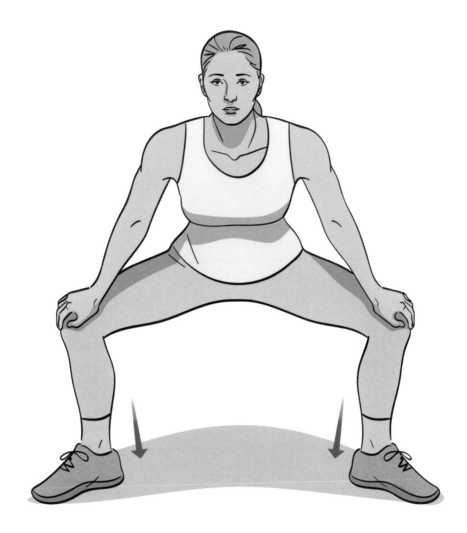

INSTRUCTIONS

1   Stand with your feet about three to four feet apart.

2   Engage your core and bend your knees, bringing your hips into a squat position with your knees in line over your ankles and your hamstrings parallel to the floor.

3   Rest your hands on your knees.

4   Hold here for 20 to 30 seconds and return to neutral position.

5   Repeat three times.

DOWNWARD DOG

AFFECTED AREAS

Buttocks: *piriformis, gluteals*

Thighs: *adductors, abductors, hamstrings*

Calves: *gastrocnemius, soleus*

Shoulders: *deltoids*

GOOD FOR

The Downward Dog is a classic, energizing yoga pose. No matter your background or age, this stretch maximizes length and strength through your entire body as you push against the floor with your arms and legs. You'll also really get your blood flowing.

LEVEL UP

For a challenge, lift your heels off the floor and come to balance on the balls of your feet. Take a slight bend in your knees, and push your hips up high and back behind you.

REMEMBER

The more firmly you push down into your heels and feet, the deeper of a stretch you will feel through your lower body and back.

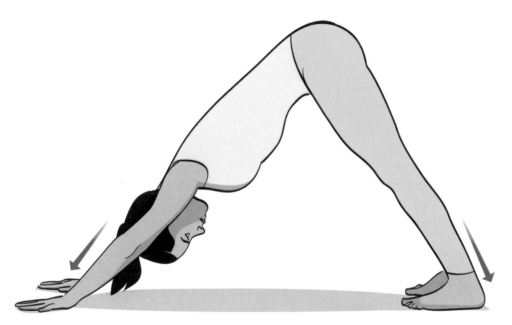

TYPE
STATIC, PASSIVE

INSTRUCTIONS

1   Kneel on all fours on a firm flat surface with your hands in line with your
    shoulders and your knees, directly below your hips.

2   Splay your fingers open, and push down into your hands and heels.
    Inhale deeply to prepare.

3   On exhale, lift your knees from the floor, straightening your legs, and
    raise your hips toward the ceiling. Think of creating a triangle shape
    with your body.

4   Engage your core, and lengthen your spine as you focus your gaze
    toward your abs.

5   Hold here 30 to 45 seconds and return to neutral position.
    Repeat twice.

WALL-ASSISTED CALF STRETCH

AFFECTED AREAS

Calves (*gastrocnemius, soleus*)
Shins (*tibialis anterior*)
Thighs (*hamstrings*)

GOOD FOR

This intense stretch for your calves and Achilles tendons is a very familiar stretch that's especially popular with runners. With the support of a wall, you can push deeper into your lower leg while maintaining your balance the entire time.

LEVEL UP

Once you've found your comfort zone in the basic calf stretch, intensify the movement by turning your feet. As you stretch your right calf, shift your toes slightly outward to the right, then to the left. You'll feel the stretch along the sides of your calf.

REMEMBER

This is a stretch that should be done gently, with little force. Take care not to overstretch your calf muscles or Achilles tendon: Press your heel down slowly each time.

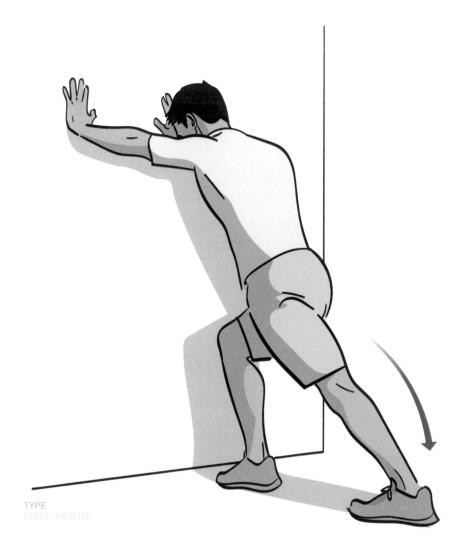

INSTRUCTIONS

1 Stand straight facing a wall or another solid surface.

2 Place your hands on the wall at shoulder height to support your weight.

3 Bend your left knee, and step your right foot back about two to three feet behind you.

4 Straighten your right knee, and press your right heel down as you gently bend your left knee deeper.

5 Hold here for 20 to 30 seconds, return to neutral position, and repeat on the opposite leg.

6 Perform three repetitions.

TOE PULL ACHILLES

AFFECTED AREAS

Calves: *gastrocnemius, soleus*
Shins: *tibialis anterior*
Thighs: *hamstrings*

GOOD FOR

This simple but intense hand-assisted stretch helps to lengthen the muscles along the back of your leg that attach from your hip and wrap down into your Achilles tendon and heel. Relieve pain in tight hamstrings and arthritic knees or ankles.

LEVEL UP

Use a resistance band to maximize the stretch in your calves and Achilles tendons. Wrap the band around the soles of your feet, and hold the ends in your hands. As you flex your feet, firmly pull against the band, and push your heels forward.

REMEMBER

Roll your shoulders back and down as you open across the front of your chest. If you need to bend your knees more to make contact with your toes, do so.

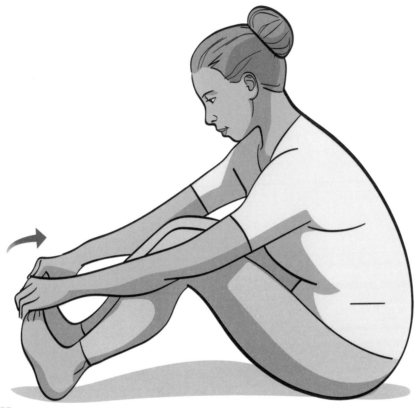

INSTRUCTIONS

1   Sit comfortably, and extend your legs straight in front of you with your legs pressed together.

2   Bend your knees as you engage your calves and flex your feet.

3   Grab hold of your toes, and pull them toward you as you push out through your heels.

4   Hold here for 10 to 20 seconds, and release to neutral position.

5   Repeat three times.

FORWARD LUNGE

AFFECTED AREAS
Thighs: *hamstrings, quadriceps, adductors*
Buttocks: *gluteals*
Shins: *tibialis anterior*

GOOD FOR

The Forward Lunge reaches deep into your hips and opens the muscles around the front and the back of your legs and pelvis. Because you need to bend deeply through your hips, be sure to thoroughly warm up your back, hips, and legs before you attempt this exercise.

LEVEL UP

Intensify the stretch by holding the lowered position for 10 to 15 seconds.

REMEMBER

Protect your knee joints by making sure that you do not overextend your front knee. As you lunge forward, your knee should extend no farther forward than your ankle.

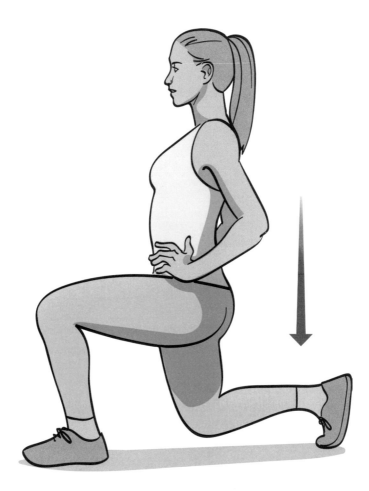

TYPE
DYNAMIC

INSTRUCTIONS

1   Begin by standing straight with your feet hip-width apart. Place your hands on your hips.

2   Step your right foot far forward, pressing down with your heel first.

3   Shift your weight over your right leg, and lower your right knee toward the floor.

4   Press your right heel into the floor to push you back to the neutral position.

5   Repeat on the opposite leg, and perform five times per side.

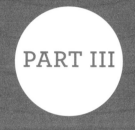

PART III

Easy Routines

EASY ROUTINES

Now that you've mastered the stretches in this book and you've built up some stamina, you can try out a few targeted routines. For easy all-around routines that are perfect for any time of day, see chapter 10, Everyday Stretches (page 162).

Need to focus on a particularly painful area of your body? Turn to chapter 11, Stretches for Aches & Pains (page 170). Here you'll find stretching routines for your back, shoulders, aching feet, and more.

Chapter 12 offers sports-specific routines (page 178) that will have you beating your competition in no time.

EVERYDAY STRETCHES

Choose from these five routines to perform every day—whether you need a routine to help you wake up in the morning or relax after a long day of work. Take a few moments between the exercises to rest, and repeat the sequences two to three times.

COMMON AREAS OF PAIN IN THE BODY

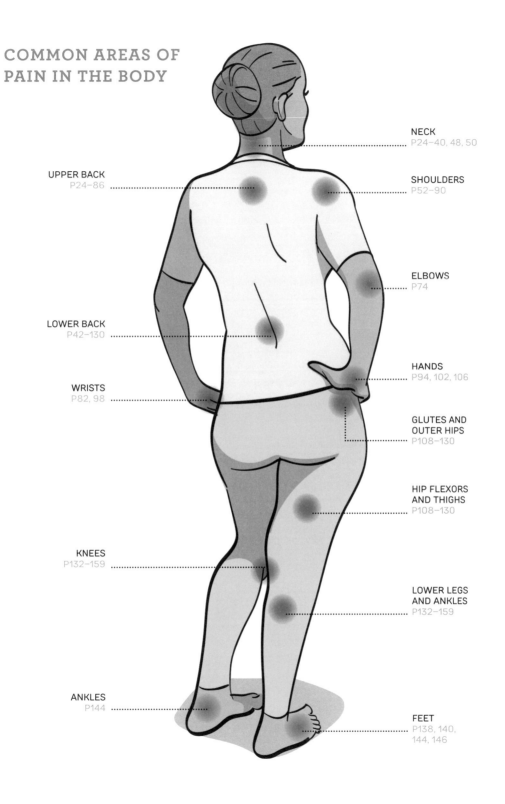

NECK
P24–40, 48, 50

UPPER BACK
P24–86

SHOULDERS
P52–90

ELBOWS
P74

LOWER BACK
P42–130

HANDS
P94, 102, 106

WRISTS
P82, 98

GLUTES AND
OUTER HIPS
P108–130

HIP FLEXORS
AND THIGHS
P108–130

KNEES
P132–159

LOWER LEGS
AND ANKLES
P132–159

ANKLES
P144

FEET
P138, 140,
144, 146

WAKING UP ROUTINE

Total time: 10 minutes

GOOD FOR

This Waking Up routine features two dynamic stretches that really get your blood flowing and two hip-flexing stretches to loosen up your lower back. It's a great way to start your day.

LEVEL UP/VARIATION

If you want to get a bit of a cardio workout, don't rest between each of the stretches but rather go directly into the next stretch.

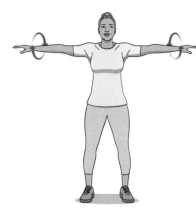

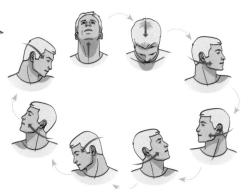

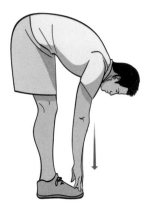

1 ARM CIRCLES
(PAGE 68)
DO FIVE REPS IN EACH
DIRECTION
DO THREE SETS

2 CERVICAL STARS
(PAGE 40)
DO THREE SETS

3 TOE TOUCH STANDING
(PAGE 132)
HOLD FOR 10 SECONDS
DO THREE SETS

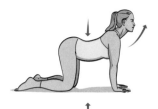

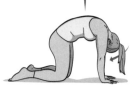

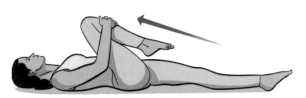

4 CAT COW
(PAGE 44)
DO 10 REPS

5 SINGLE KNEE TO CHEST
(PAGE 56)
HOLD FOR 15 SECONDS
DO THREE REPS

ENERGIZING ROUTINE

Total time: 10 minutes

GOOD FOR

If you spend long hours sitting at a desk or in a car, try this invigorating routine to loosen up your joints in your shoulders and your hips.

LEVEL UP/VARIATION

To ramp up the challenge, use light hand weights for the first and the last stretch.

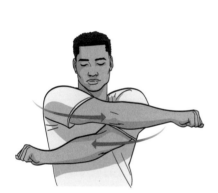

1 CRISSCROSS ARMS
(PAGE 80)
PERFORM FOR
30 SECONDS
REPEAT THREE TIMES

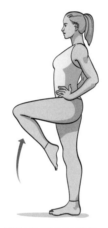

2 HIGH KNEE WALKING
(PAGE 142)
DO 10 REPS ON EACH LEG
DO THREE SETS

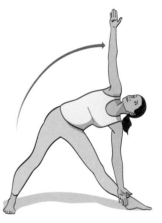

3 TRIANGLE POSE
(PAGE 120)
HOLD FOR 20 SECONDS
ON EACH SIDE
DO THREE SETS

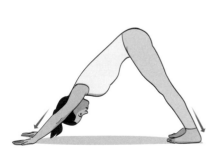

4 DOWNWARD DOG
(PAGE 152)
HOLD FOR 30 SECONDS
DO TWO SETS

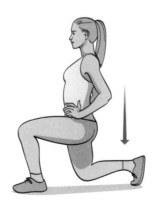

5 FORWARD LUNGE
(PAGE 158)
DO FIVE REPS ON EACH LEG
DO THREE SETS

OFFICE STRETCHES

Total time: 10 to 15 minutes

GOOD FOR

Tension can easily build up in your shoulders, back, and chest. These five stretches are a great combo for you to try anytime your upper body needs a release.

LEVEL UP/VARIATION

If you find that office work tenses up your lower back more than your upper back, add the Hip Twist or the Cobra to this routine.

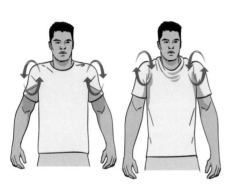

1 SHOULDER CIRCLES
(PAGE 84)
DO 10 REPS IN EACH
DIRECTION

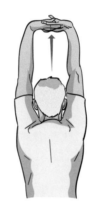

2 EXTENDED PALM PRESS
(PAGE 78)
DO FIVE REPS

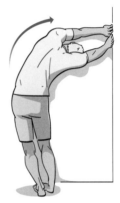

3 DOOR-ASSISTED
SIDE BEND
(PAGE 46)
HOLD FOR 30 SECONDS
REPEAT THREE TIMES

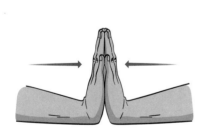

4 PRAYER HANDS
(PAGE 98)
HOLD FOR 30 SECONDS
REPEAT THREE TIMES

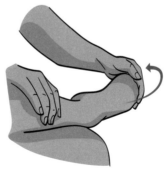

5 FOOT SICKLE
(PAGE 138)
HOLD FOR 15 SECONDS ON
EACH FOOT
DO THREE SETS

STRESS-RELEASE STRETCHES

Total time: 10 to 12 minutes

GOOD FOR

Many of us hold our tension in our necks and upper backs. To relieve some of the pent-up stress, try this routine to work out some of the kinks.

LEVEL UP/VARIATION

To reap more benefits from this sequence, try adding assisted stretches to Neck Flexion and Neck Rotation.

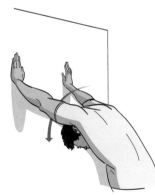

1 ELBOW CIRCLES
(PAGE 74)
DO 10 REPS IN EACH
DIRECTION

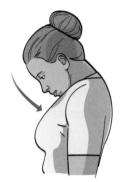

2 NECK FLEXION
(PAGE 24)
HOLD FOR 15 SECONDS
REPEAT THREE TIMES

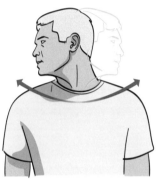

3 NECK ROTATION
(PAGE 36)
HOLD FOR 15 SECONDS
REPEAT THREE TIMES

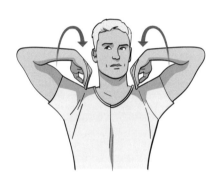

4 WALL-ASSISTED
UPPER-BACK STRETCH
(PAGE 48)
HOLD FOR 30 SECONDS
REPEAT THREE TIMES

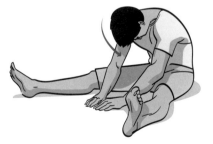

5 CENTER SPLIT
(PAGE 118)
HOLD FOR 30 SECONDS
REPEAT THREE TIMES

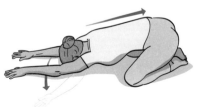

6 CHILD'S POSE
(PAGE 42)
HOLD FOR 30 SECONDS
REPEAT THREE TIMES

TECH BREAK ROUTINE

Total time: 10 to 15 minutes

GOOD FOR

High-tech devices can put a lot of strain on your upper body, arms, wrists, and fingers. This series of stretches targets these areas, which are often overused and need a little extra care.

LEVEL UP/VARIATION

If you suffer from carpel tunnel syndrome, you can add Prayer Hands (page 98) and Prayer Hands Flexion (page 100) to provide some relief for aching wrists.

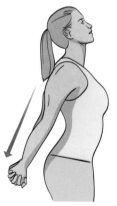

1 CERVICAL STARS
(PAGE 40)
REPEAT THREE TIMES

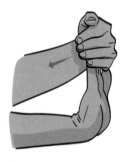

2 WRIST FLEXION
(PAGE 94)
DO 15 REPS
DO THREE SETS

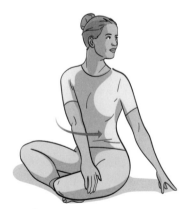

3 FINGER STRETCH
(PAGE 102)
HOLD FOR 10 SECONDS
REPEAT THREE TIMES

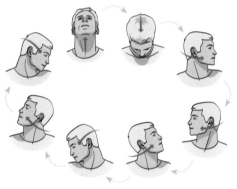

4 BENT-ARM FLY
(PAGE 72)
DO 10 REPS

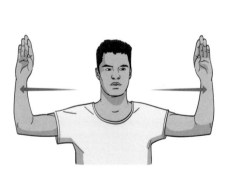

5 HANDS CLASPED
SHOULDER EXTENSION
(PAGE 76)
DO 15 REPS
DO THREE SETS

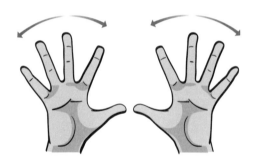

6 SEATED SPINAL TWIST
(PAGE 122)
HOLD FOR 30 SECONDS
REPEAT THREE TIMES
PER SIDE

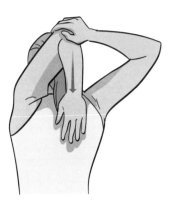

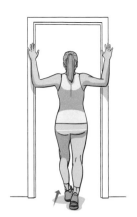

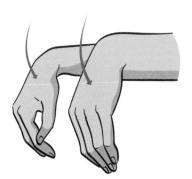

7 TRICEP STRETCH
(PAGE 90)
HOLD FOR 20 SECONDS
PERFORM THREE TIMES
ON EACH ARM

8 OPEN-DOOR PEC STRETCH
(PAGE 86)
HOLD FOR 30 SECONDS
PERFORM THREE TIMES

9 WRIST FLEXION
(PAGE 94)
HOLD FOR 10 SECONDS
REPEAT THREE TIMES

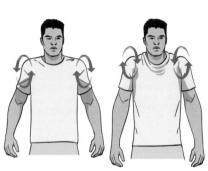

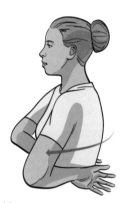

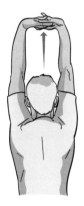

10 SHOULDER CIRCLES
(PAGE 84)
DO 10 REPS PER
DIRECTION

11 SHOULDER
HYPEREXTENSION
(PAGE 82)
HOLD FOR 30 SECONDS
REPEAT THREE TIMES

12 EXTENDED PALM PRESS
(PAGE 78)
DO FIVE REPS

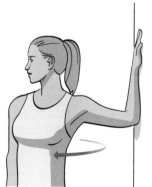

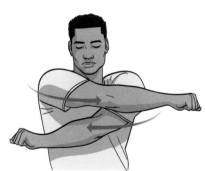

13 WALL-ASSISTED ARM
TWIST (PAGE 70)
HOLD FOR 20 SECONDS
PERFORM THREE TIMES
ON EACH ARM

14 CRISSCROSS ARMS
(PAGE 80)
PERFORM FOR
30 SECONDS
REPEAT THREE TIMES

STRETCHES FOR ACHES & PAINS

Some areas of your body may need a little extra TLC. If you suffer from tension in your shoulders or back, or if you'd like to regain mobility in your hips, try some of these targeted routines to help ease your pain.

TENSE SHOULDERS

Total time: 10 minutes

GOOD FOR

Loosen up tight shoulders and open your chest with this stress-relieving sequence. You'll improve your posture and you'll feel your upper body relax.

LEVEL UP/VARIATION

Once you have mastered this sequence, try adding the Downward Dog (page 152) at the end of the sequence to boost your energy while you stretch.

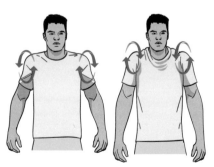

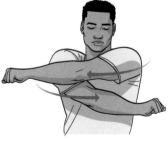

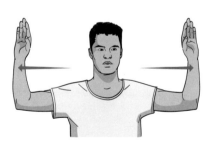

1 SHOULDER CIRCLES
(PAGE 84)
DO 10 REPS PER
DIRECTION

2 CRISSCROSS ARMS
(PAGE 80)
PERFORM FOR 30 SECONDS
REPEAT THREE TIMES

3 BENT-ARM FLY
(PAGE 72)
DO 10 REPS

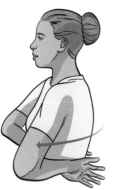

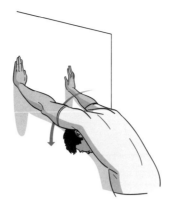

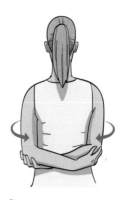

4 SHOULDER
HYPEREXTENSION
(PAGE 82)
HOLD FOR 30 SECONDS
REPEAT THREE TIMES

5 WALL-ASSISTED UPPER-
BACK STRETCH
(PAGE 48)
HOLD FOR 30 SECONDS
REPEAT THREE TIMES

6 POSTERIOR
ARM CRADLE
(PAGE 64)
HOLD FOR 30 SECONDS
REPEAT TWICE ON
EACH SIDE

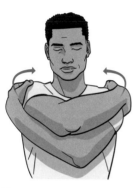

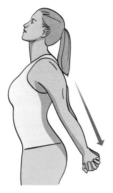

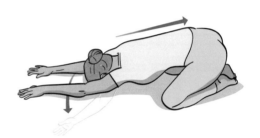

7 BEAR HUG
(PAGE 52)
HOLD FOR 20 SECONDS
REPEAT THREE TIMES

8 HANDS CLASPED
SHOULDER EXTENSION
(PAGE 76)
DO 15 REPS
DO THREE SETS

9 CHILD'S POSE
(PAGE 42)
HOLD FOR 30 SECONDS
REPEAT THREE TIMES

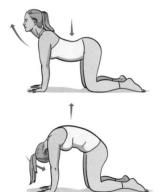

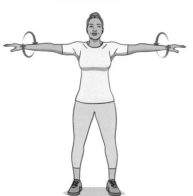

10 CAT COW
(PAGE 44)
DO 10 REPS

11 ARM CIRCLES
(PAGE 68)
DO FIVE REPS IN EACH
DIRECTION
DO THREE SETS

BACK PAIN

Total time: 12 to 15 minutes

GOOD FOR

The following sequence adds flexibility to your back, hips, abs, and glutes—all essential areas that need to be well toned for a healthy, pain-free back.

LEVEL UP/VARIATION

As you progress, increase the number of reps by one or two to gain even more benefits from this series of stretches.

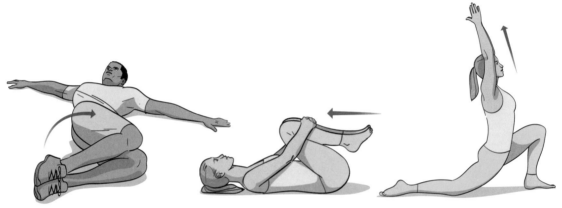

1 LOWER-BACK ROTATION
(PAGE 60)
HOLD FOR 30 SECONDS
DO THREE SETS

2 DOUBLE KNEE TO CHEST
(PAGE 58)
HOLD FOR 20 SECONDS
REPEAT THREE TIMES

3 HIP FLEXOR STRETCH
(PAGE 128)
HOLD FOR 20 SECONDS
DO THREE SETS

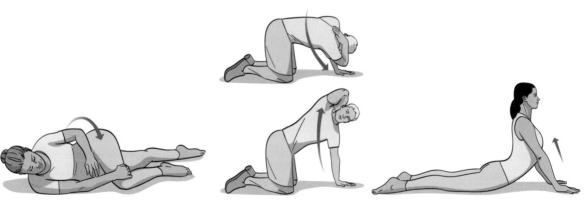

4 OPEN BOOK STRETCH
(PAGE 62)
HOLD FOR 15 SECONDS
DO THREE SETS

5 QUADRUPED ROTATIONS
(PAGE 54)
DO 10 REPS ON EACH SIDE
DO THREE SETS

6 COBRA
(PAGE 110)
HOLD FOR 30 SECONDS
REPEAT THREE TIMES

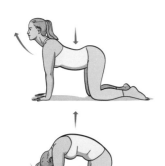

7 CAT COW
(PAGE 44)
DO 10 REPS

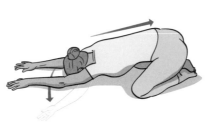

8 CHILD'S POSE
(PAGE 42)
HOLD FOR 30 SECONDS
REPEAT THREE TIMES

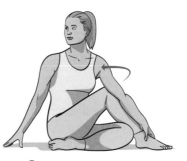

9 HIP TWIST
(PAGE 108)
HOLD FOR 20 SECONDS
REPEAT THREE TIMES
ON EACH SIDE

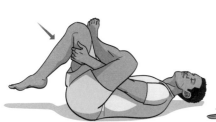

10 PIRIFORMIS STRETCH
(PAGE 114)
HOLD FOR 20 SECONDS
DO THREE SETS

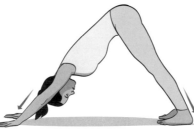

11 DOWNWARD DOG
(PAGE 152)
HOLD FOR 30 SECONDS
PERFORM TWO TIMES

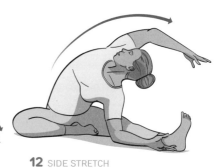

12 SIDE STRETCH
(PAGE 116)
HOLD FOR 20 SECONDS
REPEAT THREE TIMES
ON EACH SIDE

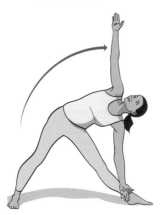

13 TRIANGLE POSE
(PAGE 120)
HOLD FOR 20 SECONDS
ON EACH SIDE
DO THREE SETS

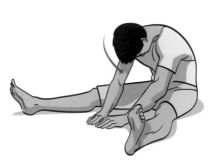

14 CENTER SPLIT
(PAGE 118)
HOLD FOR 30 SECONDS
REPEAT TWICE

HIP PAIN

Total time: 10 minutes

GOOD FOR

When one hip stretch just isn't enough, try this sequence of hip-opening exercises to really focus on the muscles in your mid-body.

LEVEL UP/VARIATION

For a dynamic variation, add Cat Cow (page 44) at the beginning of the series to wake up your whole body.

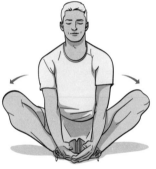

1 COBRA
(PAGE 110)
HOLD FOR 30 SECONDS
REPEAT THREE TIMES

2 BUTTERFLY
(PAGE 112)
HOLD FOR 20 SECONDS
REPEAT THREE TIMES

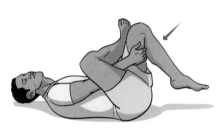

3 PIRIFORMIS STRETCH
(PAGE 114)
HOLD FOR 20 SECONDS
DO THREE SETS

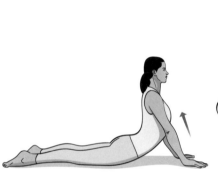

4 SIDE LUNGE
(PAGE 124)
HOLD FOR 30 SECONDS
DO THREE SETS

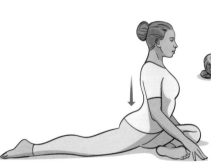

5 PIGEON POSE
(PAGE 126)
HOLD FOR 20 SECONDS
PERFORM TWICE ON
EACH SIDE

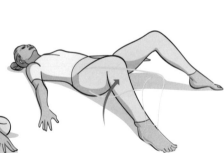

6 ALTERNATE HIP ROTATION
(PAGE 130)
DO 10 REPS ON EACH SIDE

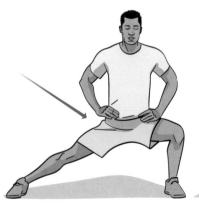

LEGS

Total time: 10 to 15 minutes

GOOD FOR

When the large muscles of your legs become tight, they benefit greatly from deep stretches that open the entire pelvic region and lengthen the muscles along the backs of your legs.

LEVEL UP/VARIATION

To increase the intensity of this series and to provide a bit of cardio, perform the stretches in quick succession, without pausing in between.

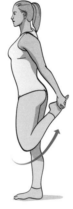

1 TRIANGLE POSE
(PAGE 120)
HOLD FOR 20 SECONDS
ON EACH SIDE
DO THREE SETS

2 STANDING QUADRICEP
STRETCH
(PAGE 134)
HOLD FOR 15 SECONDS
DO THREE SETS

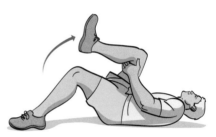

3 HAMSTRING STRETCH
(PAGE 136)
HOLD FOR 20 SECONDS
DO THREE SETS

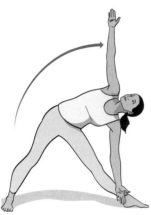

4 SUMO SQUAT
(PAGE 150)
HOLD FOR 20 SECONDS
PERFORM THREE TIMES

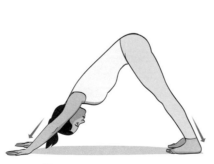

5 DOWNWARD DOG
(PAGE 152)
HOLD FOR 30 SECONDS
PERFORM TWO TIMES

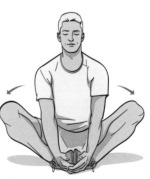

6 BUTTERFLY
(PAGE 112)
HOLD FOR 20 SECONDS
REPEAT THREE TIMES

ARMS

Total time: 10 to 15 minutes

GOOD FOR

Keep your arms and shoulders fit and toned by following this combination of static and dynamic stretches.

LEVEL UP/VARIATION

When you're ready, increase the level of difficulty in this series by adding light wrist weights.

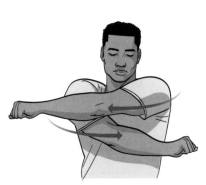
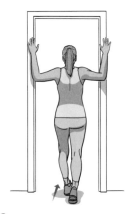
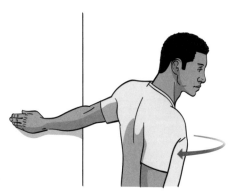

1 CRISSCROSS ARMS
(PAGE 80)
PERFORM FOR
30 SECONDS
REPEAT THREE TIMES

2 OPEN-DOOR PEC STRETCH
(PAGE 86)
HOLD FOR 30 SECONDS
PERFORM THREE TIMES

3 WALL-ASSISTED BICEP STRETCH
(PAGE 88)
HOLD FOR 30 SECONDS
PERFORM THREE TIMES
ON EACH ARM

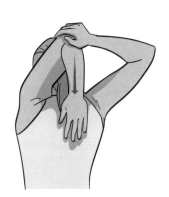
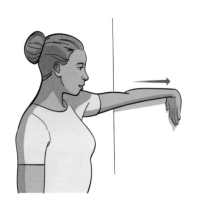
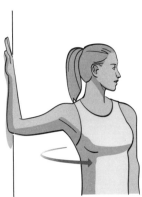

4 TRICEP STRETCH
(PAGE 90)
HOLD FOR 20 SECONDS
PERFORM THREE TIMES
ON EACH ARM

5 WALL-ASSISTED FOREARM
STRETCH (PAGE 96)
HOLD FOR 20 SECONDS
PERFORM THREE TIMES
ON EACH ARM

6 WALL-ASSISTED ARM TWIST
(PAGE 70)
HOLD FOR 20 SECONDS
PERFORM THREE TIMES
ON EACH ARM

CHEST

Total time: 10 minutes

GOOD FOR

This sequence helps you to open your chest and improve your breathing and circulation.

LEVEL UP/VARIATION

Challenge yourself by holding each stretch for a longer duration, but remember to breathe throughout.

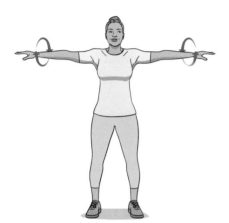

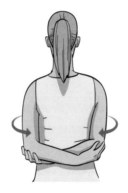

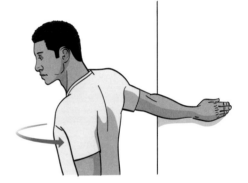

1 ARM CIRCLES
(PAGE 68)
DO FIVE REPS IN EACH
DIRECTION
DO THREE SETS

2 POSTERIOR ARM CRADLE
(PAGE 64)
HOLD FOR 30 SECONDS
REPEAT THREE TIMES

3 WALL-ASSISTED BICEP STRETCH
(PAGE 88)
HOLD FOR 30 SECONDS
PERFORM THREE TIMES
ON EACH ARM

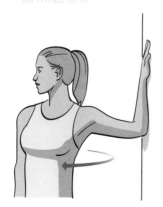

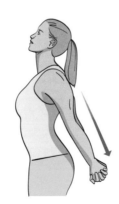

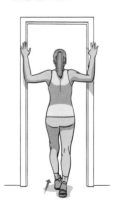

4 WALL-ASSISTED ARM TWIST
(PAGE 70)
HOLD FOR 20 SECONDS
PERFORM THREE TIMES
ON EACH ARM

5 HANDS CLASPED
SHOULDER EXTENSION
(PAGE 76)
DO 15 REPS
DO THREE SETS

6 OPEN-DOOR PEC STRETCH
(PAGE 86)
HOLD FOR 30 SECONDS
PERFORM THREE TIMES

CHAPTER 12

ACTIVITY-SPECIFIC STRETCHES

To help you prepare for your favorite activity or sport, check out some of these routines. You'll be able to warm up the appropriate muscles and keep them toned and ready for action.

BIKING

Total time: 10 to 12 minutes

GOOD FOR

Tone your arms and lengthen your glutes, thighs, and calves with these biker-friendly stretches.

LEVEL UP/VARIATION

Balance your muscles groups by stretching your upper body. Add dynamic Arm Circles (page 68) and your favorite shoulder stretches to keep your whole body well toned.

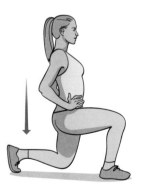

1 FORWARD LUNGE
(PAGE 158)
DO FIVE REPS ON
EACH LEG
DO THREE SETS

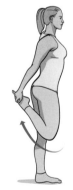

2 STANDING QUADRICEP
STRETCH
(PAGE 134)
HOLD FOR 15 SECONDS
DO THREE SETS

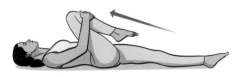

3 SINGLE KNEE TO CHEST
(PAGE 56)
HOLD FOR 15 SECONDS
REPEAT THREE TIMES ON
EACH LEG

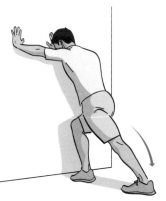

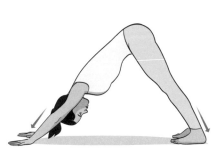

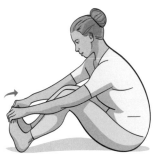

4 WALL-ASSISTED CALF
STRETCH
(PAGE 154)
HOLD FOR 20 SECONDS
REPEAT THREE TIMES

5 DOWNWARD DOG
(PAGE 152)
HOLD FOR 30 SECONDS
PERFORM TWO TIMES

6 ACHILLES TOE PULL
(PAGE 156)
HOLD FOR 20 SECONDS
PERFORM THREE TIMES

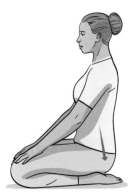

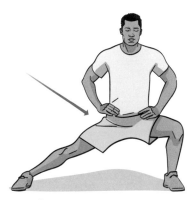

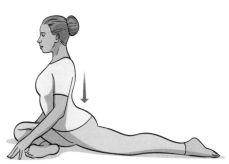

7 TIBIALIS KNEE STRETCH
(PAGE 148)
HOLD FOR 30 SECONDS
REPEAT THREE TIMES

8 SIDE LUNGE
(PAGE 124)
HOLD FOR 30 SECONDS
PERFORM THREE SETS

6 PIGEON
(PAGE 126)
HOLD FOR 20 SECONDS
REPEAT TWICE ON
EACH SIDE

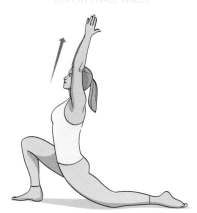

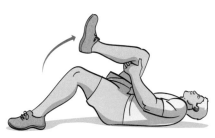

7 HIP FLEXOR STRETCH
(PAGE 128)
HOLD FOR 20 SECONDS
PERFORM THREE SETS

8 HAMSTRING STRETCH
(PAGE 136)
HOLD FOR 20 SECONDS
REPEAT THREE TIMES ON
EACH LEG

RUNNING/WALKING

Total time: 15 minutes

GOOD FOR

Get ready to hit your stride with this sequence, which focuses on the major leg muscles and joints.

LEVEL UP/VARIATION

Try adding light ankle weights to increase the challenge as you perform the leg stretches.

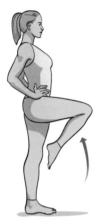
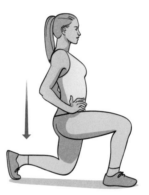
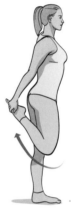

1 HIGH KNEE WALKING
(PAGE 142)
DO 10 REPS ON EACH LEG
DO THREE SETS

2 FORWARD LUNGE
(PAGE 158)
DO FIVE REPS ON EACH LEG
DO THREE SETS

3 STANDING QUADRICEP
STRETCH
(PAGE 134)
HOLD FOR 15 SECONDS
DO THREE SETS

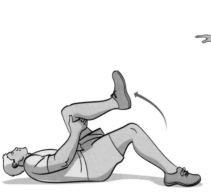
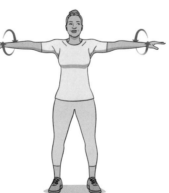
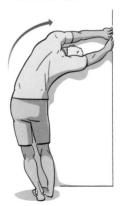

4 HAMSTRING STRETCH
(PAGE 136)
HOLD FOR 20 SECONDS
DO THREE SETS

5 ARM CIRCLES
(PAGE 68)
DO FIVE REPS IN EACH
DIRECTION
DO THREE SETS

6 DOOR-ASSISTED
SIDE BEND
(PAGE 46)
HOLD FOR 30 SECONDS
REPEAT THREE TIMES

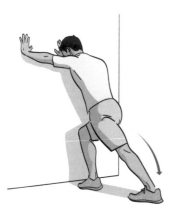
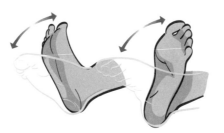
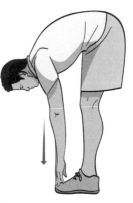

7 WALL-ASSISTED CALF
STRETCH
(PAGE 154)
HOLD FOR 20 SECONDS
REPEAT THREE TIMES

8 POINTE AND FLEX
(PAGE 146)
HOLD FOR 10 SECONDS IN
EACH DIRECTION
REPEAT THREE TIMES

9 TOE TOUCH STANDING
(PAGE 132)
HOLD FOR 10 SECONDS
PERFORM THREE SETS

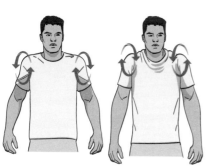
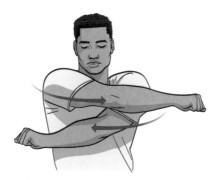
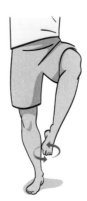

10 SHOULDER CIRCLES
(PAGE 84)
DO 10 REPS PER
DIRECTION

11 CRISSCROSS ARMS
(PAGE 80)
PERFORM FOR
30 SECONDS
REPEAT THREE TIMES

12 ANKLE CIRCLES
(PAGE 144)
REPEAT FIVE TIMES
ON EACH FOOT

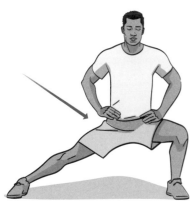
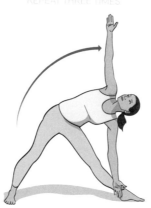
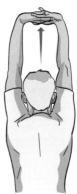

13 SIDE LUNGE
(PAGE 124)
HOLD FOR 30 SECONDS
PERFORM THREE SETS

14 TRIANGLE POSE
(PAGE 120)
HOLD FOR 20 SECONDS ON
EACH SIDE
DO THREE SETS

15 EXTENDED PALM PRESS
(PAGE 78)
DO FIVE REPS

DRIVING

Total time: 10 minutes

GOOD FOR

What is worse than getting to your destination after a long drive and feeling knotted up and achy? This sequence will ease your stiff joints and aching back.

LEVEL UP/VARIATION

Don't wait until you reach your destination to stretch. Pull over during your drive and run through some of these stretches to ease discomfort.

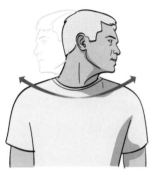

1 NECK ROTATION
STRETCH
(PAGE 36)
HOLD FOR 15 SECONDS
DO THREE SETS

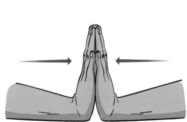

2 PRAYER HANDS
(PAGE 98)
HOLD FOR 30 SECONDS
PERFORM THREE TIMES

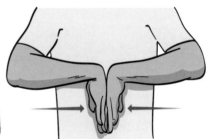

3 PRAYER HANDS FLEXION
(PAGE 100)
HOLD FOR 20 SECONDS
PERFORM THREE TIMES

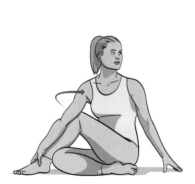

4 HIP TWIST
(PAGE 108)
HOLD FOR 20 SECONDS
REPEAT THREE TIMES ON
EACH SIDE

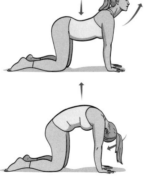

5 CAT COW
(PAGE 44)
PERFORM 10 REPS

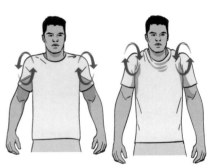

6 SHOULDER CIRCLES
(PAGE 84)
PERFORM 10 REPS PER
DIRECTION

SWIMMING

Total time: 7 to 10 minutes

GOOD FOR

Be sure to warm up your shoulders, arms, and legs with this series of stretches before you start doing your laps in the pool.

LEVEL UP/VARIATION

Consider using light hand weights to strengthen your upper while you stretch.

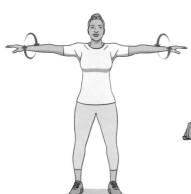
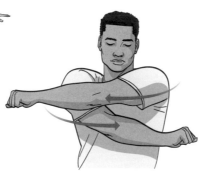
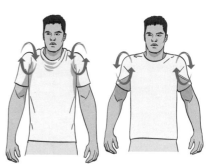

1 ARM CIRCLES
(PAGE 68)
DO FIVE REPS IN EACH
DIRECTION
DO THREE SETS

2 CRISSCROSS ARMS
(PAGE 80)
PERFORM FOR 30 SECONDS
REPEAT THREE TIMES

3 SHOULDER CIRCLES
(PAGE 84)
DO 10 REPS PER
DIRECTION

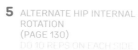
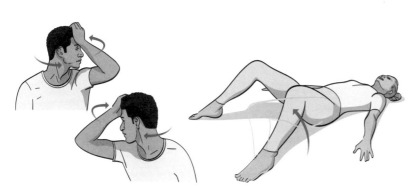
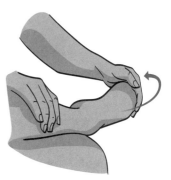

4 NECK ROTATION
ASSISTED
(PAGE 38)
HOLD FOR 15 SECONDS
DO THREE SETS

5 ALTERNATE HIP INTERNAL
ROTATION
(PAGE 130)
DO 10 REPS ON EACH SIDE

6 FOOT SICKLE
(PAGE 138)
HOLD FOR 15 SECONDS
PERFORM THREE TIMES
ON EACH FOOT

TENNIS

Total time: 10 minutes

GOOD FOR

Quick reflexes on the court start with toned, flexible limbs and a stable, balanced core, which these stretches help provide.

LEVEL UP/VARIATION

For a more dynamic take on this series, add High Knees Walking (page 142) at the beginning of the series.

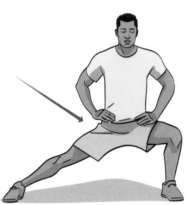

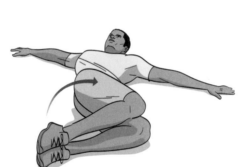

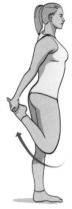

1 SIDE LUNGE
(PAGE 124)
HOLD FOR 30 SECONDS
DO THREE SETS

2 LOWER-BACK ROTATION
(PAGE 60)
HOLD FOR 30 SECONDS
DO THREE SETS

3 STANDING QUADRICEP
STRETCH
(PAGE 134)
HOLD FOR 15 SECONDS
DO THREE SETS

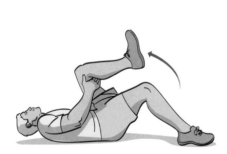

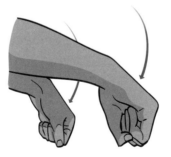

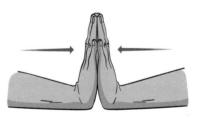

4 HAMSTRING STRETCH
(PAGE 136)
HOLD FOR 20 SECONDS
DO THREE SETS ON
EACH LEG

5 FIST ROTATION
(PAGE 104)
DO FIVE ROTATIONS IN EACH
DIRECTION FOR EACH FIST
DO THREE SETS

6 PRAYER HANDS
(PAGE 98)
HOLD FOR 30 SECONDS
PERFORM THREE TIMES

WEIGHT TRAINING

Total time: 12 to 15 minutes

GOOD FOR

Stabilize your legs and core as you strengthen and tone your upper body with these effective stretches.

LEVEL UP/VARIATION

Add the challenging Center Split (page 118) to this series for a deep hip-opening and increased mobility in your hips.

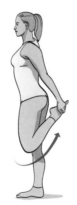 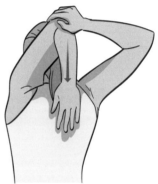 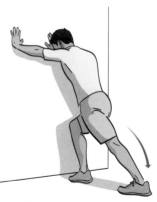

1 OPEN-DOOR PEC STRETCH (PAGE 86)
HOLD FOR 30 SECONDS
PERFORM THREE TIMES

2 WALL-ASSISTED BICEP STRETCH (PAGE 88)
HOLD FOR 30 SECONDS
PERFORM THREE TIMES ON EACH ARM

3 TRICEP STRETCH (PAGE 90)
HOLD FOR 20 SECONDS
PERFORM THREE TIMES ON EACH ARM

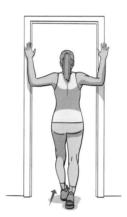 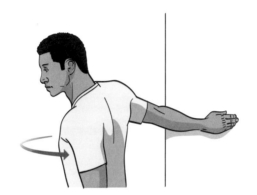 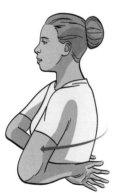

4 SHOULDER HYPEREXTENSION (PAGE 82)
HOLD FOR 30 SECONDS
REPEAT THREE TIMES

5 QUADRICEP STRETCH (PAGE 134)
HOLD FOR 15 SECONDS
DO THREE SETS

6 WALL-ASSISTED CALF STRETCH (PAGE 154)
HOLD FOR 20 SECONDS
REPEAT THREE TIMES

RESOURCES

The following books, organizations, and their websites serve as trusted resources for providing further information on stretching and general health and fitness.

BOOKS

Arming, Phil and Michael A. Martyn. *Stretching for Functional Flexibility*. Baltimore: Lippincott Williams & Wilkins, 2010.

Liebman, Hollis. *1,500 Stretches: The Complete Guide to Flexibility and Movement*. New York, Black Dog & Leventhal, 2017.

Matthews, Jessica. *Stretching to Stay Young: Simple Workouts to Keep You Flexible, Energized, and Pain Free*. Althea Press, 2016.

Nelson, Arnold G. and Jouko Kokkonen. *Stretching Anatomy*, 2nd ed. Chicago: Human Kinetics, 2014.

Albir, Guillermo Seijas. *Anatomy and 100 Essential Stretching Exercises*. Hauppauge, New York: Barrons Educational Series, 2015.

ORGANIZATIONS & WEBSITES

American College of Sports Medicine: ASCM.org

National Academy of Sports Medicine: NASM.org

National Strength and Conditioning Association: NSCA.com

United States Registry of Exercise Professionals: USreps.org

ENDNOTES

CHAPTER 1

1. Cho, Sung-Hak and Soo-Han Kim. "Immediate Effect of Stretching and Ultrasound on Hamstring Flexibility and Proprioception." *Journal of Physical Therapy Science*, vol. 28, no. 6 (June 2016): 1806–1808. DOI: 10.1589/jpts.28.1806

2. Wong, Alexei and Arturo Figueroa. "Effects of Acute Stretching Exercise and Training on Heart Rate Variability: A Review," *Journal of Strength and Conditioning Research* (February 2019). DOI: 10.1519/JSC.0000000000003084

3. Reddy, Ravi Shankar and Khalid A Alahmari. "Effect of Lower Extremity Stretching Exercises on Balance in Geriatric Population." *International Journal of Health Sciences*, vol. 10, no. 3 (July 2016): 389–395. PMCID: PMC5003582

4. Edeer, Ayse, Allison Licardo, Alanna Rooney, Danielle Freund, and Valerie Olson. "The Effects of Static Versus Dynamic Stretching on Average Power in The Young-Adult Athletic Population." *MOJ Yoga and Physical Therapy*, vol. 1, no. 1 (2016): 25–30. DOI: 1.10.15406/mojypt.2016.01.00006

5. Kim, Giwon, Hyangsun Kim, Woo K Kim, and Junesun Kim. "Effect of Stretching-Based Rehabilitation on Pain, Flexibility and Muscle Strength in Dancers with Hamstring Injury: A Single-Blind, Prospective, Randomized Clinical Trial." *The Journal of Sports Medicine and Physical Fitness*, vol. 58, no. 9 (October 2017): 1287–1295. DOI: 10.23736/S0022–4707.17.07554–5

6. Dantas, Estélio H.M., Estevão Scudese, Rodrigo G.S. Vale, Gilmar W. Senna, Ana Paula de A. Albuquerque, Olívia Mafra, Fabiana R. Scartoni, Mario Cezar S. Conceição. "Flexibility Adaptations in Golf Players During a Whole Season," *Journal of Exercise Physiology Online*, vol. 21, no. 2 (April 2018): 193–201. https://www.researchgate.net/publication/324074773_Flexibility_Adaptations _in_Golf_Players_during_a_Whole_Season

INDEX

ACKNOWLEDGMENTS

Many thanks and gratitude to my family, friends, and partner Eddy for their ever-encouraging love and support. Dr. Phil Striano, you are so much fun! Thank you for sharing this book together with me.

Audra Avizienis, beautiful and generous woman, thank you for your epic work within these pages. And thank you Sean Moore, Moseley Road, and Callisto for the opportunity to create this wonderful book for the world.

May the love and energy that I put into this book go out into the world and serve as a tool for personal growth, healing, and self-care for others.

—Natasha Diamond-Walker

Since 1994, I have had the distinct privilege of treating thousands of individuals from many different walks of life. Healing people and helping them return to their daily activities—from grandparents playing with their grandchildren to athletes getting back on the field to workers returning to their jobs—has been incredibly rewarding for me.

I want to take this opportunity to thank my parents, Drs. Philip and Theresa Striano, for guiding me through the years to get to this point in my life. Dad, although my time with you was short, your sacrifice for, and conviction in, your profession, patients, and family will always be a guiding force for me. I also want to acknowledge my three sisters, Terri, Thomasina, and Tara, for their love and support.

My two boys, Christian and Brandon, you two fill my life with joy and pride—I love you both with all my heart. Shelly and Stacy, thank you both for these two divine gifts.

I am grateful to my co-author, Natasha Diamond-Walker, for your many contributions to this book. It was a pleasure collaborating with you.

Finally, I am deeply indebted to Moseley Road editorial director Audra Avizienis, without whom this book would not have been possible. I am truly grateful for your invaluable insight, skillful guidance, and unwavering support throughout this project.

—Philip Striano, DC

ABOUT THE AUTHORS

Natasha Diamond-Walker was born and raised in Los Angeles, California. She is an internationally recognized dancer and actress who currently performs as a Soloist with the Martha Graham Dance Company in New York City. Natasha has worked extensively in TV, film, theater, and live performance venues. Drawing upon her background in the arts, dance, health, and wellness, she has discovered a passion for writing. She is a Fordham University/Ailey School alumna.

Philip Striano, DC is the owner of Hudson Rivertown's Chiropractic Health Care in Dobbs Ferry, New York. He is a certified chiropractic sports physician and a specialist in sports injury, exercise, and strength and conditioning. He received his doctor of chiropractic degree from New York Chiropractic College. He is a lifelong resident of Irvington, New York, where he lives with his two sons, Christian and Brandon.